Clinical Assessment Skills

for Physiotherapists

and Occupational Therapists | Allied Health Professionals

A Comprehensive Guide to Physical Diagnosis

- Subjective and Neurological Assessment
- Assessment of Higher Function
- Cranial Nerve and Sensory Assessment
- Reflex Examination
- Motor Examination
- Gait Assessment
- ADL Assessment
- Bldder and Bowel Assessment
- Balance and Coordination

- Psychological Assessment
- Musculoskeletal Assessment
- Goniometry
- Limb Length and Girth Measurement
- Special Tests in Musculoskeletal Assessment
- Obstetrics and Gynecology Assessment
- Pediatric Assessment
- Cardiorespiratory Assessment
- Laboratory Investigations

Clinical Assessment Skills

for Physiotherapists

and Occupational Therapists | Allied Health Professionals

A Comprehensive Guide to Physical Diagnosis

Gowrishankar Potturi PhD (PT), MIAP

Lecturer, Paramedical Vigyan Mahavidyalaya, Saifai, Etawah, UP
Ex-Faculty, AUCMS, Malaysia.

KB Ranjeet Singh Chaudhary BPT, MPT (Ortho), MIAP

Demonstrator, Paramedical Vigyan Mahavidyalaya, Saifai, Etawah, UP

Neha Rastogi BPT, MPT (Neuro), MIAP

Demonstrator, Paramedical Vigyan Mahavidyalaya, Saifai, Etawah, UP

Anjali Agarwal BPT, MPT (Neuro), MIAP, BEd (Spl. Ed), Dip. Yoga, Dip. Nutrition and Dietetics

Demonstrator, Paramedical Vigyan Mahavidyalaya, Saifai, Etawah, UP

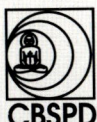

CBSPD

CBS Publishers & Distributors Pvt Ltd

New Delhi • Bengaluru • Chennai • Kochi • Kolkata • Lucknow • Mumbai
Bhopal • Bhubaneswar • Hyderabad • Jharkhand • Nagpur • Patna • Pune • Uttarakhand

Clinical Assessment Skills
for Physiotherapists
and Occupational Therapists | Allied Health Professionals
A Comprehensive Guide to
Physical Diagnosis

ISBN: 978-93-86217-61-5

First Edition: 2017
   Reprint: 2020, 2023, 2024, 2025

Published by Satish Kumar Jain and produced by Varun Jain for
CBS Publishers & Distributors Pvt Ltd
4819/XI Prahlad Street, 24 Ansari Road, Daryaganj, New Delhi 110 002, India.
Ph: 23289259, 23266861   Website: www.cbspd.com
                                 e-mail: delhi@cbspd.com

Corporate Office: 204 FIE, Industrial Area, Patparganj, Delhi 110 092, India.
Ph: 4934 4934   Fax: 4934 4935   e-mail: publishing@cbspd.com; publicity@cbspd.com

Branches

- **Bengaluru:** Seema House 2975, 17th Cross, KR Road, Banasankari 2nd Stage, Bengaluru 560 070, Karnataka, India
  Ph: +91-80-26771678/79   Fax: +91-80-26771680   e-mail: bangalore@cbspd.com
- **Chennai:** 7, Subbaraya Street, Shenoy Nagar, Chennai 600 030, Tamil Nadu, India
  Ph: +91-44-26680620, 26681266   Fax: +91-44-42032115   e-mail: chennai@cbspd.com
- **Kochi:** 42/1325, 36, Power House Road, Opposite KSEB, Kochi 682 018, Kerala, India
  Ph: +91-484-4059061-67   Fax: +91-484-4059065   e-mail: kochi@cbspd.com
- **Kolkata:** C/o Hind Ceramics Compound, 1st Floor, 147, Nilgunj Road, Belghoria, Kolkata 700 056, West Bengal, India
  Ph: +91-33-25633055/56   e-mail: kolkata@cbspd.com
- **Lucknow:** Basement, Khushnuma Complex, 7-Meerabai Marg (behind Jawahar Bhawan), Lucknow 226 001, Uttar Pradesh, India
  Ph: +91-522-4000032   e-mail: tiwari.lucknow@cbspd.com
- **Mumbai:** PWD Shed, Gala No. 25/26, Ramchandra Bhatt Marg, Next to JJ Hospital Gate No. 2, Opp Union Bank of India, Noorbaug, Mumbai 400 009, Maharashtra, India
  Ph: +91-22-66661880/89   e-mail: mumbai@cbspd.com

Representatives

- **Hyderabad**   0-9885175004   - **Jharkhand**   0-9811541605   - **Nagpur**   0-8692091830
- **Patna**   0-9334159340   - **Pune**   0-9664372571   - **Uttarakhand**   0-9716462459

Printed at: HT Media Ltd., Greater Noida, UP, India.

to

Our Director

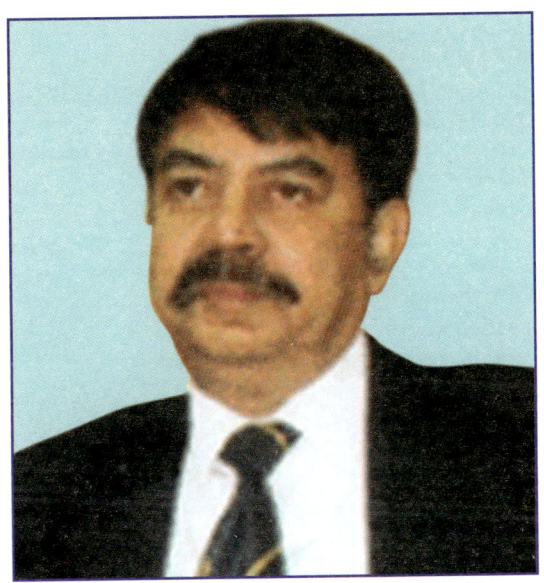

Dr (Brig) T Prabhakar VSM

MBBS, MD, PDCC (Neuroanesthesia)

Preface

The skill of assessment for any health care professional is vital as it gives the pathway to diagnosis and further plan the treatment. There are a few books available today for training assessment to physiotherapists. The idea beyond the introduction of this book is to give a comprehensive idea on clinical assessment to various areas of physiotherapy. Almost all the main clinical areas of interest of the physiotherapists are included in this book.

The book is designed to suit the students and professionals of physiotherapy. Care is taken to incorporate most of the assessment skills without overburdening. The book is expected to be useful to the students of occupational therapy and allied health sciences also. The language is kept as simple as possible.

We hope this book will be helpful to guide you not only to get success in the examinations but also in your clinical career.

Particular effort has been made to avoid mistakes but if found and brought to our notice, will be corrected in the next edition.

Gowrishankar Potturi
KB Ranjeet Singh Chaudhary
Neha Rastogi
Anjali Agarwal

Acknowledgments

We render our regards to:

- Dr T Prabhakar, Director, UPRIMSNR, Saifai, Etawah, UP
- Dr Arun Nagrath, Principal, Paramedical Vigyan Mahavidyalaya, Saifai, Etawah, UP
- Dr Suraj Kumar, Head, Department of Physiotherapy, Paramedical Vigyan Mahavidyalaya, Saifai, Etawah.

Picture courtesy:
- Mr Devesh
- Mr Sher Mohammad
- Mr Asif
- Mr Amar Kushwaha
- Mr Subhashchandra
- Mr Gaurav Dubey

Gowrishankar Potturi
KB Ranjeet Singh Chaudhary
Neha Rastogi
Anjali Agarwal

Contents

Preface vii

Acknowledgments viii

1. Introduction to Assessment and Diagnosis 1

2. Subjective Assessment 2

3. Neurological Assessment 4

4. On Observation in Neurological Cases 9

5. On Palpation in Neurological Cases 10

6. Assessment of Higher Function 12

7. Cranial Nerve Assessment 14

8. Sensory Assessment 25

9. Reflex Examination 30

10. Motor Examination 38

11. Gait Assessment 42

12. Bladder and Bowel Assessment 46

13. ADL Assessment 47

14. Psychological Assessment 48

15. Balance and Coordination 49

16. Musculoskeletal System Assessment 52

17. Measurement of Range of Motion (Goniometry) 53

18. Limb Length Measurements 62

19. Limb Girth Measurements — 64

20. Common Special Tests in Musculoskeletal Assessment — 67

21. Obstetrics and Gynecology Assessment — 79

22. Pediatric Assessment — 81

23. Cardiorespiratory Assessment — 93

Cardiopulmonary Assessment Form   93
Observation Skills in Cardiopulmonary Cases   97
On Palpation in Cardiopulmonary Cases   101
Tracheal Shift/Mediastinal Shift   102
Vocal Fremitus   103
Examination of the Distal Pulses   103
Recording of Arterial Blood Pressure   106
Assessment of Jugular Venous Pressure   107
Apex Heart Beat   108
Examination of Chest Shape and Dimensions   108
Examination of Breathing Pattern   109
Examination of Chest Mobility   110
Percussion   111
Auscultation Skills   112
Examination of Cough   113
Target Heart Rate   114

24. Investigations — 115

Examination of a Chest Radiograph   115
Basics of Electrocardiogram (ECG)   122
Electrodiagnosis SD Curve   130
FG Test   132
Nerve Conduction Velocity   134
Electromyography   136
CT Scan (Computerised Tomography Scan)   138
Magnetic Resonance Imaging (MRI)   142
How to Check the BMI (Body Mass Index)?   147
Manual Muscle Testing   148

Index — 165

Introduction to Assessment and Diagnosis

A clinical assessment usually involves conducting examination and gathering the information that makes a clinician to determine a diagnosis.

DIAGNOSIS

The act or process of identifying or determining the nature and cause of a disease or injury through evaluation of patient history, examination and review of laboratory data.

Need of Diagnosis

- Diagnosis is a very important tool for identifying the underlying medical problem of the patient.
- It helps in identifying the problem and helps in proper planning of the treatment.
- It helps in identifying the prognosis of the disease.

The clinical assessment usually involves questioning, observing and examining the client about the nature, duration and severity of the client's problems.

A good assessment should cover the client's all possible physical assessment.

The assessment usually contains two basic areas:

1. Subjective assessment
2. Objective assessment

A *subjective assessment* is a method of documentation about the patient by directly asking the patient or relatives or obtaining from the clinical data, e.g. admission Notes.

An *objective assessment* is one in which the clinician shall perform various skills to identify the pathology that lead to the chief complaint/s of the patient.

2

Subjective Assessment

Name: Patient's name indicates his/her identity. It is helpful in easy search among several patients, e.g. if two patients are admitted of same age, they can be differentiated by their names.

Age: Patient's age determine his/her condition among patient's having same name.

It also helps a medical professional to reach a diagnosis and prognosis of the condition, e.g. osteoarthritis or osteoporosis is common in older individuals than the young patients. Whereas Scheuermann's disease is common in youngs.

Gender: It determines the identity of the patient. It is also helpful in determining the prevalence of condition which are more common to gender specific, e.g. anaemia frequently more prevalent in females than in males.

Occupation: Occupation of a patient determines the disease suffered since long time he/she is in that occupation, e.g. a person who is field labour is likely to develop muscle strain than a person who is computer operator will suffer from a neck pain.

Address: This helps in finding a patient's locality. It is an important part of patient's subjective history. Address of a patient determines about a disease/condition's prominancy, e.g. patient belonging to a particular area may be more prone to malaria than some areas more prominent for water diseases.

Dominant side: Right- or left-handed

IP no./hospital no. This is an unique number given to a patient who is admitted to the hospital. It is written on the patient's file. This is known as in-patient number or hospital number.

This number bears every information regarding the concerned patient. When a patient is admitted to the same hospital for the same or different condition, this number may be accessed to gather his/her previous information. This number may contain serial number, date, month, year, any alphabet, e.g. IP no as 786-08-08-2015AC

Referral: Patient when given first aid and further medical facility is not available at that centre, he/she is referred to a hospital where better treatment and care can be provided, e.g. a patient who suffered a severe head injury in a road traffic accident (RTA) was taken to a clinic where first aid and dressing was available. After dressing and first aid, patient is referred to hospital by the doctor.

Date of admission:

Date of evaluation:

Chief complain: These are the main problems faced by the patient when admitted to the hospital. These are written by the medical person in patient's own words in chronological order; that is major problems come first. Medical terminologies shouldn't be used. Chief complains can be gathered directly from the patient or can be from patient's attendant.

History

This means the events took place from starting of the condition till present. This can be gathered directly through the patient or through the attendant.

Present History

It describes patient's condition in chronological order.

- Mode of onset—sudden or gradual condition/disease is suddenly appeared or appeared slowly.
- Mechanism of injury.
- Through what way patient was injured. While gathering the information, the examiner should determine the magnitude and direction of the injuring force.
- Symptoms that make patient uneasy, restless in day or night or throughout 24 hours.
- *Relieving/aggravating factors:* Activities which give relief and activities which increase the condition.
- *Duration/period:* Time from when he/she suffering the condition. If the condition started initially, it is acute or if it is of longer duration, it is chronic in nature.
- *Treatment/medication*: If received, record it, mention the dosage, procedure, timing.
- Patient whether conscious or not when came to the treatment centre/hospital, e.g. patient was apparently well till this afternoon 12/01/1999, when he met with a road traffic accident while driving the motorcycle. He was hit by a truck from back. He was thrown onto the side of the road with severe injury to pelvic region. He became unconscious and was brought to a near by clinic where first aid was given and referred to AIIMS. X-ray and other investigations were done. He was diagnosed with fracture hip bone and was operated for the same. Medication and physiotherapy are given as per the orders.

Past History

This detail about any history of the same or other condition which the patient met earlier, e.g. patient suffered from an RTA in which he had fractured his right radius ulna around 10 years back.

Medical History

Means any history of medical problems and any previous surgeries the patient undergone of any region of the body and its medication if presently continuing, should be in knowledge of the examiner. This helps the examiner to take care while prescribing any exercises or investigation.

Personal History

This indicates patient's personal habits like chewing tobacco, smoking, alcohol consumption, or any habits which are hindering his/her health, e.g. if a person smokes, then this is harmful for his lungs, may result in lung disease.

Marital Status

If a patient is married, then his/her partner can look after the patient by giving physical and mental support.

Family History

This means whether patient have a nuclear or joint family. It includes the spouse, children in a nuclear family, or children, mother, father or any other members in a joint family.

In a joint family, patient receives a better care and treatment than the nuclear family due to more no of family members.

Economic History

This indicates the economic status of the patient. How much is the income, its source and how much is the expenditure. It plays an important role in his/her rehabilitation, e.g. if patient is a poor man, he will not be able to take adequate treatment due to lack of funds.

Therapist has to design treatment plan according to the fund available with the patient or relatives.

Social History

This deals with patient's social and education status.

Social status: Social status means patient's self presentation in society.

- Does patient like to meet people in the surroundings?
- Does he respect and understand the values of other individuals?
- Whether he/she adapts among many people?

Education status: If patient is educated, he/she will be able to communicate politely with others and judge them.

3

Neurological Assessment

SUBJECTIVE

Name   :
Dominance   :
Address   :
Socioeconomic status   :
Age   :
Sex   :
Occupation   :
Chief complaints   :
   According to the chronological order
   (Major problems come first)

… … … … … … … … … … … … …
… … … … … … … … … … … … …
… … … … … … … … … … … … …

… … … … … … … … … … … … …

HISTORY

Past Medical History

Any previous history of same problem

Present Medical History

Onset   : (Sudden/gradual)
Duration   :
Side   :
Associated problem   : Problems other than the
                    primary one

Personal History

Family History

OBJECTIVE ASSESSMENT

On Observation

Posture

Levels of ear   : Equal/unequal
Levels of shoulder   : Equal/unequal
Levels of ASIS   : Equal/unequal

Gait

Normal/Abnormal

External Appliances

- Splints
- Braces
- Bandages

On Palpation

Muscle tone   : Increased/decreased
Skin temperature
Abnormal prominence

Edema

Location/generalized/localized/pitting/
nonpitting/endurated/non-endurated

On Examination

Vital signs

Blood pressure   : (120/80 mm Hg)
Temperature   : (98.6°F)
Respiratory rate   : (16–18 cycles/minute)
Heart rate   : (72–80 beats/minute)

HIGHER FUNCTION

Level of Consciousness

Glasgow Coma Scale

- Eye opening
  - ↳ None—even to pain
  - ↳ To pain—pain from stimulus to limbs
  - ↳ To speech—opens eyes on verbal approach
  - ↳ Spontaneous—opens eye spontaneously
- Motor response
  - ↳ None—to any pain, limbs remain flaccid
  - ↳ Extension to pain—shoulder adducted/internally rotated, forearm pronated.
  - ↳ Abnormal flexion to pain—shoulder flexes/adducts
  - ↳ Flexion/withdrawal to pain—(flexion of elbow, supination of forearm, flexion of wrist when supraorbital pressure applied; pulls part of body away when nailbed pinched
  - ↳ Localizes pain—arm attempts to remove supraorbital pain
  - ↳ Obeys commands—follows command.
- Verbal response
  - ↳ None—as stated
  - ↳ Incomprehensive—moaning but no words
  - ↳ Inappropriate—random or exclamatory articulated speech, but no conversational exchange.
  - ↳ Confused—the patient responds to questions coherently but there is some disorientation and confusion.
  - ↳ Oriented—patient responds coherently and appropriately to questions such as the patient's name and age, where they are and why, the year, month, etc.)

Scoring

Eye opening	4
Motor response	6
Verbal response	5
Total	15

Generally, brain injury is classified as:
- Severe, with GCS ≤8—that is also a generally accepted definition of a coma
- Moderate, GCS 9–12
- Minor, GCS ≥13.

Memory

i. Instant
ii. Short term
iii. Long term

Intelligence

Checked by simple mathematical calculations

Behaviour

Orientation

i. By place
ii. By time
iii. By person

Speech

Identify for any speech disorder related to neurological imbalance.

CRANIAL NERVE ASSESSMENT

Sensory Assessment

Superficial

- Pain
- Touch
  - ↳ Fine
  - ↳ Crude
- Temperature

Deep

- Pressure
- Vibrations
- Joint Position sense
- Joint Kinesthetic sense

Combined Cortical Sensation

- Tactile localization
- Stereognosis (object recognition)
- Two-point discrimination

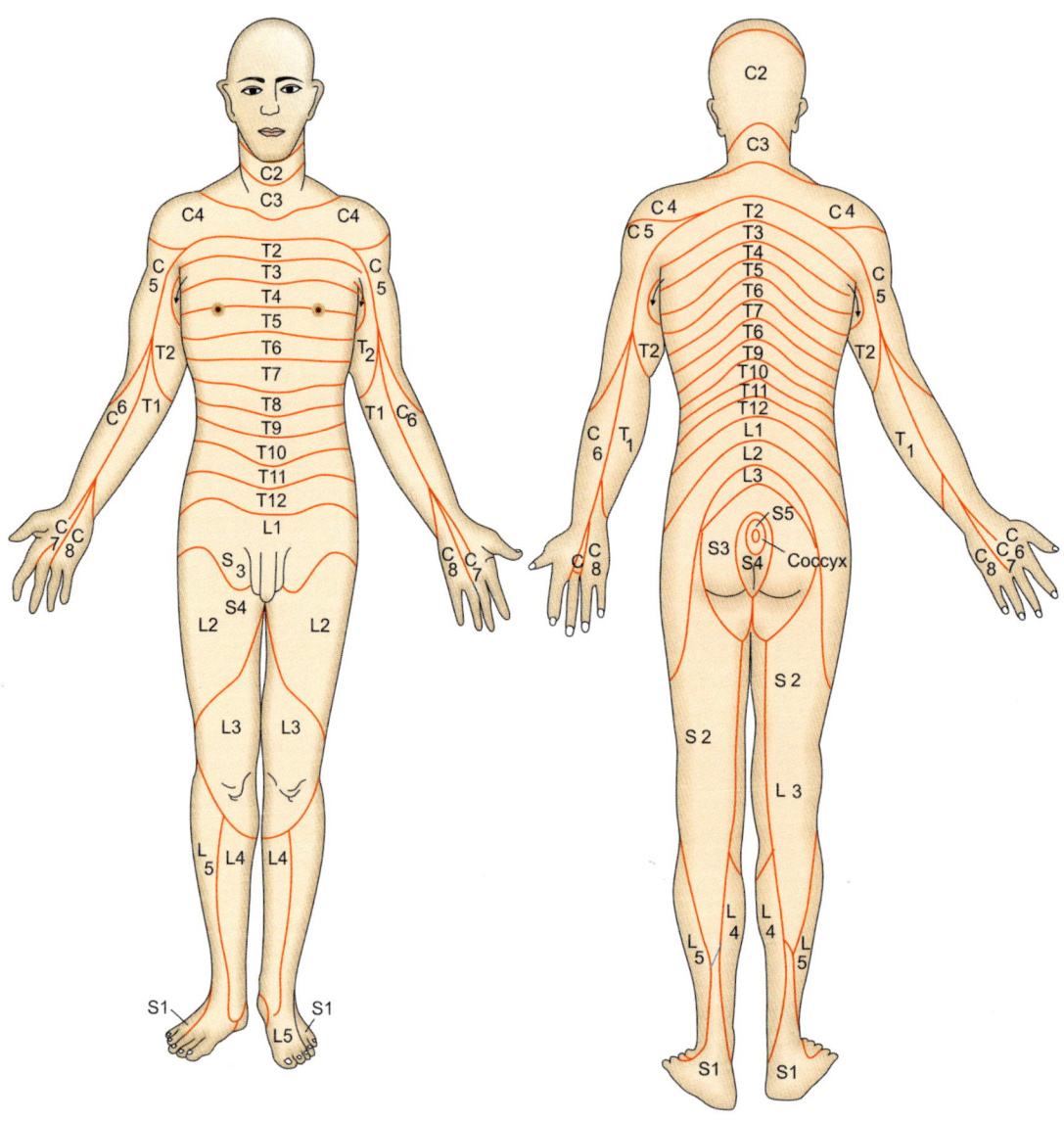

REFLEX EXAMINATION

Superficial

- Corneal reflex
- Pupillary reflex
- Gag reflex
- Abdominal reflex
- Cremastric reflex
- Plantar / babinski

Deep

- Biceps jerk
- Triceps jerk
- Brachioradialis jerk
- Knee jerk
- Ankle jerk

Grades

0   —   No response
1+ —   Depressed
2+ —   Average
3+ —   Brisker than normal
4+ —   Very brisk or hyperactive

MOTOR ASSESSMENT

Tone

Muscle tone

+2	Spasticity
+1	Hypertonicity
0	Normal
-1	Hypotonicity
-2	Flaccidity

Modified Ashworth scale for grading spasticity

Grade	Description
0	No increase in muscle tone.
1	Slight increase in muscle tone, manifested by a catch and release, or by minimal resistance at the end of the ROM when the affected part(s) is moved in flexion or extension.
2	Slight increase in muscle tone, manifested by catch, followed by minimal resistance throughout the remainder (less than half) of the ROM.
3	More marked increase in muscle tone through most of ROM.
4	Considerable increase in muscles tone, passive movement difficult.
5	Affects part(s) rigid in flexion or extension.

Spasticity

Characteristics of spasticity:

1. *Clasp-knife reflex:* An initial high resistance followed by a sudden relaxation or letting go of a spastic muscle in response to a stretch reflex.
2. *Clonus:* Cyclic hyperactivity of antagonistic muscles occurring at a regular frequency in response to sustained stretch to a spastic muscle.

Muscle Power

Based on MRC grading

0 No contraction
1 Flicker of contraction
2 Able to do the movement in gravity eliminated plane
3 Able to do the movement against gravity
4 Able to do the movement against gravity with minimal resistance
5 Able to do the movement against gravity with maximal resistance

Myotomes

Voluntary Control

Voluntary control grades

Grade 0 = No flicker of contraction

Grade 1 = Flicker of contraction/initiation of movement in pattern or synergy

Grade 2 = Half range of motion in synergy/pattern

Grade 3 = Full range of motion in pattern/synergy

Grade 4 = Initial half range on isolation and later half in pattern/synergy

Grade 5 = Full range of motion on isolation but goes into pattern/synergy on resistance

Grade 6 = Full range of motion on isolation against resistance

Balance Test

Normal : Patient able to maintain steady balance without handhold support.

Good   : Patient able to maintain balance without handhold support, limited postural sway.

Fair   : Patient able to maintain balance with handhold support, may require occasional minimal assistance.

Poor   : Patients require handhold support and moderate to maximal assistance to maintain position.

Berg Balance Scale Score

Gait assessment: Normal/abnormal

Trendelenburg sign

The trendelenburg sign is said to be positive if, when standing on one leg, the pelvis drops on the side opposite to the stance leg. The weakness is present on the side of the stance leg.

Scissor gait

Walk like X, because of the tightness of adductors of hip.

Antalgic gait

The individual favors certain motions to avoid acute pain.

Festinating gait

The patient moves with short, jerky steps.

Drunken sailor gait (cerebellar ataxia)

Characterised by uncertain start and stop, lateral deviations, and unequal steps.

Waddling gait

Walk like a duck, swaying of trunk either side because of the paralysis of hip abductors on both sides.

High stepping gait

Walk on forefoot, because of paralysis of dorsiflexors.

Gluteus maximus gait

The patient do back sway to compensate the weakness.

ADL Assessment

Ambulation   : Dependent/Independent
Bathing   : Dependent/Independent
Communication   : Dependent/Independent
Dressing   : Dependent/Independent
Eating   : Dependent/Independent

SPECIAL TESTS

Related to condition

....

DIAGNOSIS

X-ray   : Findings
CT scan   : Findings
MRI   : Findings

MEDICAL TREATMENT

Wincosin
Gait assessment scale   :
Coordination   :
Bowel and bladder   :
Psychological assessment :

PHYSIOTHERAPY TREATMENT

Aims (Chronological Order)

To......................................
To......................................
To......................................

Means

Modalities
Exercises
And Etc.....

4

On Observation in Neurological Cases

ON OBSERVATION

- The neurological assessment helps to find out, how much the patient improves and how much the condition deteriorates. These data are recorded for systemic observations.
- These observations are best performed in altered or impaired level of consciousness.
- A well-trained staff/faculty in theory and practical are needed to perform these neurological observations.

ON EXAMINATION

Posture and Attitude

The position of all limbs and posture of the patient needs to be examined and noticed.

Wasting

Muscle wasting is most commonly seen in lower motor neuron lesion. There should be a proper specification of muscles that are wasted in comparison with the non-affected side. In upper motor neuron disease (chronic conditions), wasting is most commonly seen because of disuse of the part.

Examination: Compare the affected side with the non-affected one.

Result: Change in the muscle girth visually.

- Look for any extraneous movements: Fasciculations or twitches, etc.
- Look for speed of movements, e.g. bradykinesia.

Tropic Changes

- Observe the shape, symmetry and size of the muscle.
- Check for any hypertrophy, atrophy or abnormal bulging or depression.

- Check for any rashes, spots, nail brittleness, Dry scaly skin or erythema, etc.

Involuntary Movements

Involuntary movements include fasciculations, tics, dystonia, chorea, athetosis, etc.

- *Fasiculation*: Muscle quivering under skin.
- *Tics:* The contraction in which single or group of muscles are involuntary contracted resulting in stereotyped movements.
- *Dystonia:* Slow sustained abnormal movements.
- *Chorea:* Irregular repetitive jerky movements.
- *Athetosis*: Irregular repetitive writhing movements.

Speech

The speaking capability of a patient is checked like:

- *Dysarthria*: In this condition, there is a problem with articulation with retained comprehension due to weakness of orolingual muscles. The speech construction is normal. Ask a patient to speak 'WEST REGISTER STREET'.
- *Dysphonia*: In this condition, patient has hoarseness of voice due to laryngeal problems.
- *Dysphasia*: Receptive dysphasia is difficulty in comprehension, while expressive dysphasia is difficulty in putting words together to make meaning. This is due to a lesion in the language areas of the dominant hemisphere.

Gait

- In this we have to check for the walking pattern of the patient when they enter the room and check for the evidence of hemiparesis, foot drop, ataxic gait, Parkinson's gait, etc.

5

On Palpation in Neurological Cases

Palpate the supraclavicular fossae and look for enlarged lymph nodes or cervical ribs.

Inpect the several individual muscles to see for muscle wasting, hypertrophy, or fasciculations and in cases f suspected myositis just palpate the affected site of the muscles to see if there is tenderness.

Tenderness is graded as:

1. *Severe:* If patient shows grimace on face with touch
2. *Moderate*: If patient shows grimace on face to HOLD
3. *Mild*: If patient shows grimace on face to PRESS.

Note: The examiner should never ask the patient about the experience of pain during checking of tenderness, but should identify by facial expressions of the patient.

ASSESSMENT OF EDEMA

Edema

Technique for evaluation of edema

1. Examiner impresses thumb into skin over bony surface:
   - Tibia
   - Fibula
   - Sacrum
2. Withdraw thumb
3. Measure depth of pit and record in millimeters check for the edema and report it as follows:
   - *Location of edema*: Precisely locate the anatomical position of the edema, e.g. *a localized edema on the dorsum of right forearm.*

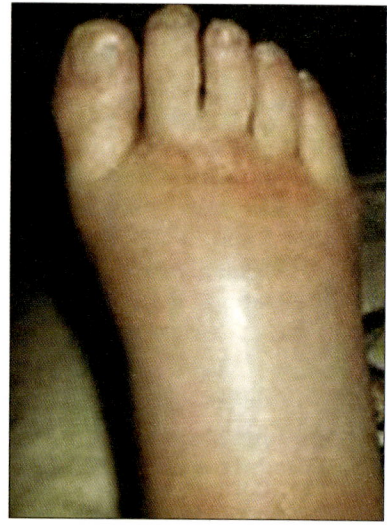

Indurated edema

- *Indurated or non-indurated*: Indurated edema will be hard and firm and non movable, i.e. it will not be able to drain physically by maneuvers like effleurage
  - Non-indurated edema will be movable and could be drained by physical maneuvers like effleurage.
  - Indurated edema can be due to local trauma, inflammation or infection
  - It can be seen bilaterally in cases of heart diseases, renal dysfunction, abdominal mass, lung dysfunctions.
- *Pitting or non-pitting*: If there is a observable swelling over the body tissues due to fluid accumulation and when a pressure is applied over the area, if

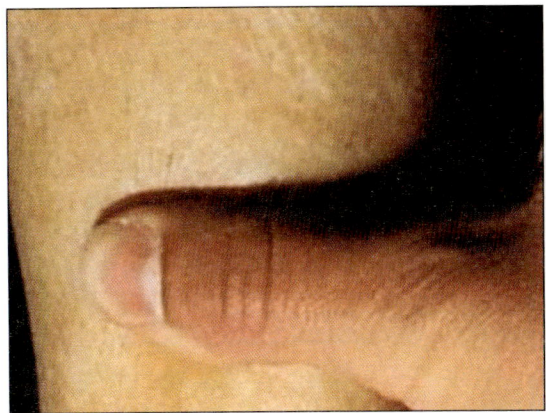
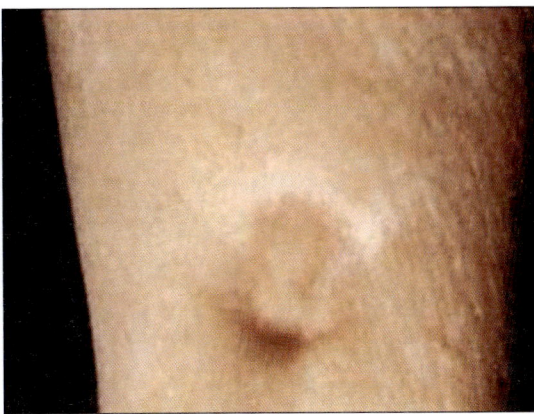

Pitting type edema

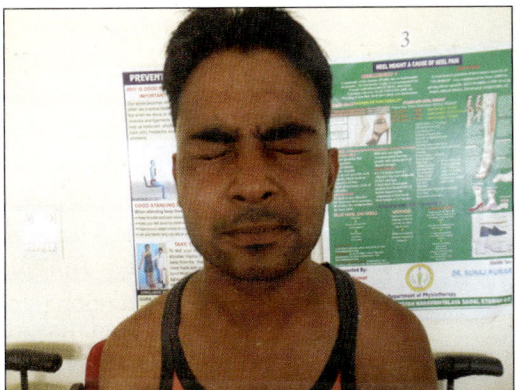

Grimace

there is an indentation that persists for sometime after the release of pressure, it is called pitting edema.

➲ It is commonly seen in systemic diseases like hypertension.

➲ If there is no indentation seen after the pressure is released, then it is non-pitting.

↳ *Localized or generalized:* If there is swelling observed on a precise area, it is localized and if there is a gross swelling, then it is called as generalized.

6

Assessment of Higher Function

LEVEL OF CONSCIOUSNESS

Glasgow Coma Scale

Activity	Score
• **Eye opening**	
Spontaneous	4
To speech	3
To pain	2
No response	1
• **Best motor response**	
Follows motor commands	6
Localizes	5
Withdraws	4
Abnormal flexion	3
Extensor response	2
No response	1
• **Verbal response**	
Oriented	5
Confused conversation	4
Inappropriate words	3
Incomprehensible sounds	2
No response	1
Total	**15**

Generally, brain injury is classified as:

- *Severe* : GCSd ≤8 (generally, accepted definition of coma)
- *Moderate* : GCS 9–12
- *Mild* : GCSe ≥13

Higher Function

1. Attention
2. Memory
3. Calculation
4. Abstract thought
5. Spatial
6. Visual and body perception
7. Apraxia

Attention and Orientation

Orientation is tested by questioning on time, place and person.

- *Time*: Day, date, month, year, season, time of day.
- *Place*: City, hospital, birth place of him.
- *Person*: His name, job, etc.
    - ✎ Make a note of errors made by the patient.
    - ✎ Attention is tested by using digit span, by noting the number of digits the patient is able to recall forwards and backwards but not repeated digits as 333.
    - ✎ Normal digit span is seven forwards and five backwards.

Memory

a. *Immediate recall and attention*: By name and address test.
(*Note*: Number of errors in repeating the name and address and after how many attempts it is repeated clearly.)
b. *Short-term memory*: After 5 minutes, again ask the patient to repeat the name and address used in immediate recall.
c. *Long-term memory*: In this, test factual knowledge, e.g. first prime-minister of India

Calculation

To be tested by simple mathematical calculations.

Abstract Thought

This is used to test frontal lobe function. This is done by:

- Asking the patient to explain well-known proverbs.
- Asking the patient to explain the difference between pairs of objects, e.g. a table and a chair.
- Asking the patient to estimate.

Spatial

This is used to test parietal and occipital lobe function, also for dementias.

- Clock face (patient is asked to draw a clock with the given time).
- Five-pointed star (patient is asked to copy a five-pointed star).

Interpretation

- Accurate clock and star: Normal response.
- Half clock missing: Visual inattention.
- Unable to draw clock or reproduce star: Constructional apraxia.

Visual and Body Perception

Test for parietal and occipital lesions.

- *Facial recognition*: Ask the patient to identify 'Famous faces'.
- *Body perception*: Ask the patient to touch or point out the parts of his body as asked.
- *Sensory agnosia*: Ask the patient to close his eyes and write a letter or number on his hand and ask what it is and place an object in his hand and ask him what it is.

Apraxia

Inability to perform a task when there is no weakness or movement disorder or inco-ordination to prevent it.

- Ask the patient to perform an imaginary task.
- Ask the patient to copy your hand movements.

7

Cranial Nerve Assessment

There are 12 pairs of cranial nerves present in human beings. Cranial nerves constitute a part of peripheral nervous system. The cranial nerves in craniological order are as follows:

    I. Olfactory
   II. Optic
  III. Oculomotor
  IV. Trochlear
   V. Trigeminal
  VI. Abducens

   VII. Facial
  VIII. Vestibulocochlear
    IX. Glossopharyngeal
     X. Vagus
    XI. Spinal accessory
   XII. Hytpoglossal

One or more nerves can be affected depending on the cause, e.g. space occupying lesions (SOL), mysthenia gravis, multiple sclerosis, etc.

The cranial nerves are tested as given in figure below.

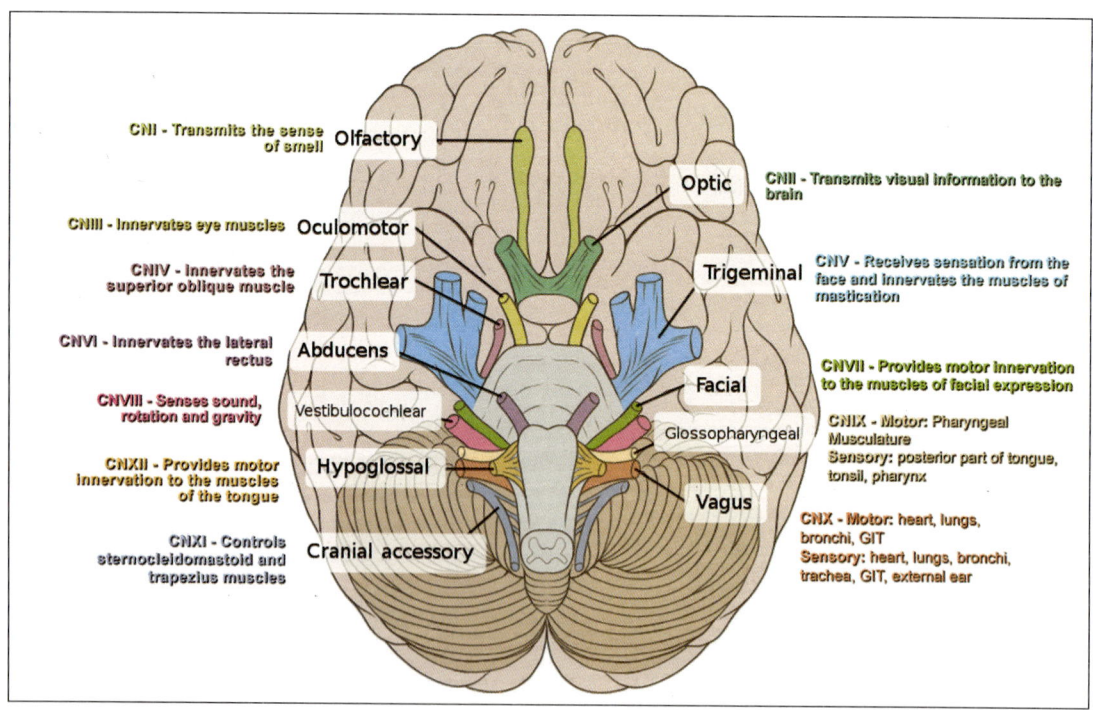

OLFACTORY NERVE

The main function is smell.

Procedure

1. Wash your hands properly. Introduce yourself to the patient.
2. Explain the procedure clearly and in a simple way to obtain consent of the patient.
3. Make the patient sit in front of you with eyes closed.
4. Ask the patient to close one nostril.
5. Now offer something familiar to the patient to smell and identify by keeping the object 10 cm away from the nostril.
6. Usually, a lemon peel, garlic, ginger, coffee can be offered.
7. Now ask the patient to close the other nostril and identify the smell.

Loss of smell is called as anosmia.

Interpretation

1. If the patient is able to identify, the olfactory is functioning normal.
2. If the patient is unable to identify, then the following can be the reasons.

   a. Prior upper respiratory infections.
   b. Head injuries.
   c. Nasal and paranasal sinus disease causing damage to olfactory neuroepithelium.
   d. Neurodegenerative diseases.
   e. Iatrogenic interventions, e.g. septoplasty, rhinoplasty, radiation therapy, etc.
   f. Intracranial tumors or intranasal neo-plasms.
   g. Epilepsy, hypothyroidism, renal diseases.
   h. Some studies have shown that loss of smell is seen in disorders associated with cerebellar degeneration, e.g. Friedreich's ataxia.
   i. It is a hallmark sign in schizophrenia.
   j. Some cases of migraine.
   k. Viral infections.

OPTIC NERVE

It is the second cranial nerve. It is a sensory nerve and is mainly involved for vision. The optic nerve is tested for

a. Acuity of vision
b. Colour vision
c. Field of vision
d. Pupillary reflex
e. Fundoscopy examination

Acuity of Vision

- The acuity of vision is tested with the help of Snellen's chart.
- The normal acuity of vision is 6/6 or 20/20 in humans.
- If the patient wears glasses or contact lens normally, then the test must be checked with and without vision aids and report separately.
- If you are checking a hand-held Snellen's chart, then hold the chart at a 14 inches distance from the patient. Hold the chart at the level of eye of the patient.
- Ask the patient to close one eye each time and read aloud the smallest letter they are able to see.
- If you are using a wall mounted Snellen's chart, then the distance between the patient and the chart should be 20 feet.

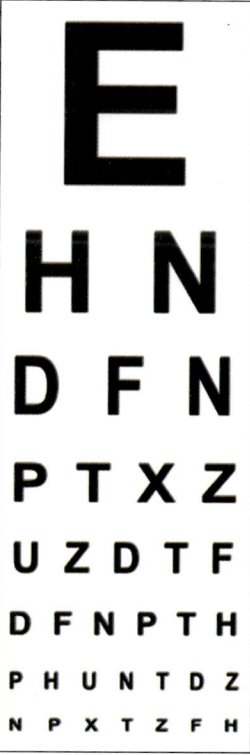

Interpretation

- Visual acuity is expressed as a fraction.
- The numerator or the top number refers to the distance you stand from the chart.
- The denominator or bottom number indicates the distance at which a person with normal eye sight could read the same line you correctly read.
- For example, 20/20 is considered to be normal in humans. A 20/40 reading reports that the patient could correctly read at 20 feet away which can be read by a person with normal vision from 40 feet away .
- If the patient can't identify all items correctly, number missed is listed after a "–" sign, e.g. 20/80–2 for 2 missed on 20/80 line .

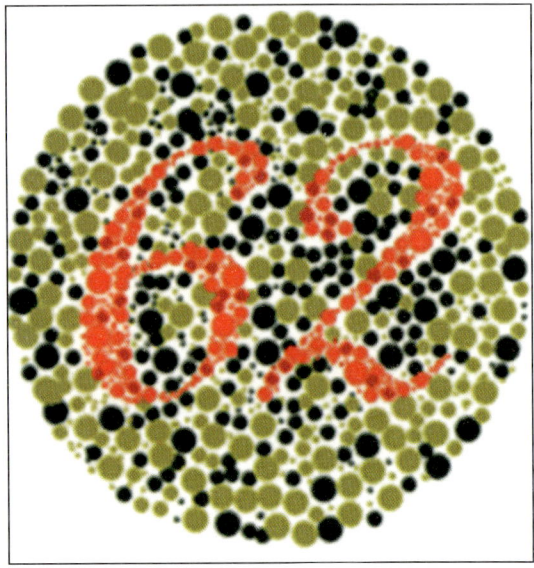

Colour Vision

- Colour vision is tested using Ishihara plates which help to identify the patients who are colour blind.
- This test is the most widely accepted test and used for testing red-green colour vision deficiency and contains 38 plates of circles created by irregular coloured dots in two or more colours.
- The patient is asked to close one eye for testing and vice versa.
- The plates are kept in front of the patient and will be asked to identify the number on the plate.

Field of Vision

Visual fields are tested by asking the patient to look directly at you while you wiggle one of your fingers in each of the four quadrants of visual field of each eye.

Hemianopia is the blindness of the half of the visual field.

The most common causes are stroke, brain trauma or tumor.

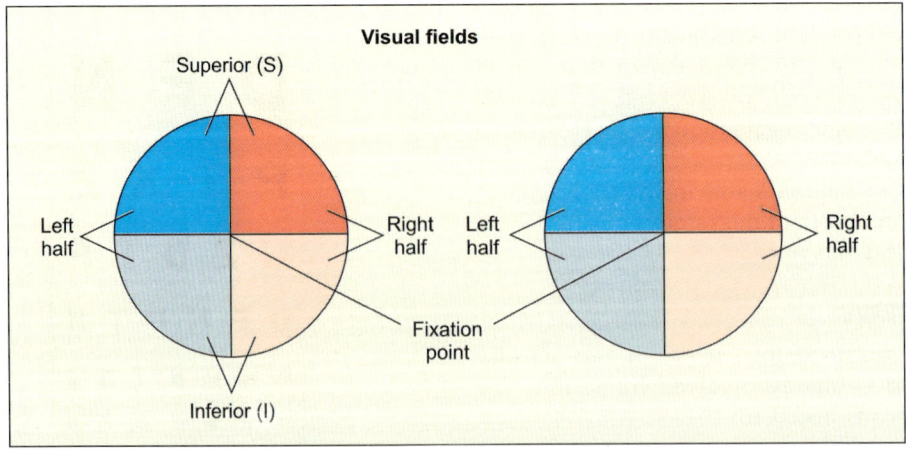

Procedure

- Face the patient approximately 1–2 feet apart.
- Close your right eye and ask the patient to close his/her left eye.
- Move your left arm out and away keeping it at equal distance from both of you.
- Rise your index finger, such that it should be just outside your field of vision.
- Wiggle the index finger and bring it in towards the noses. You and your patient should be able to detect it at the same time.
- Repeat the moving finger in each direction. Use other hand to check the medial field, starting in front of the closed eye.
- Repeat the entire procedure for the other eye as well.

Pupillary Reflex

The pupillary reflex involves adjustments in pupil sizes with changes in the intensity of light.
The optic nerve is involved in the pupillary reflex.

Procedure

- Make sure that the room is dark and pupils are dilated a little.
- The room should not be completely dark that you can't observe the pupil reaction.
- Make the patient sit calmly on a chair and ask him to look straight.

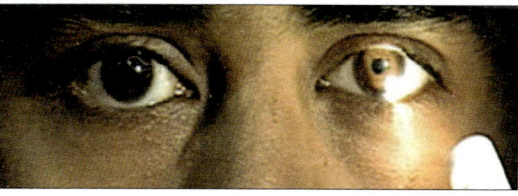

- Now shine the light in right eye and observe the pupil being constricted.
- Now repeat the same procedure on left eye.

Interpretation

- Usually the normal response of pupillary reaction is described as "PERRLA" (pupils equal, round, reactive to light accommodation).
- Abnormal responses are observed secondary to direct or indirect damage to optic nerve,

parasympathetic injury or to the sympathetic neurons.
- Some sympathomimetics, like cocaine, will dilate the pupil and some narcotics, like heroin, will constrict the pupil.

Fundoscopy

Fundoscopy also known as ophthalmoscopy is a test that allows a health professional to see inside the fundus of the eye and other structures using an ophthalmoscope or fundoscope.

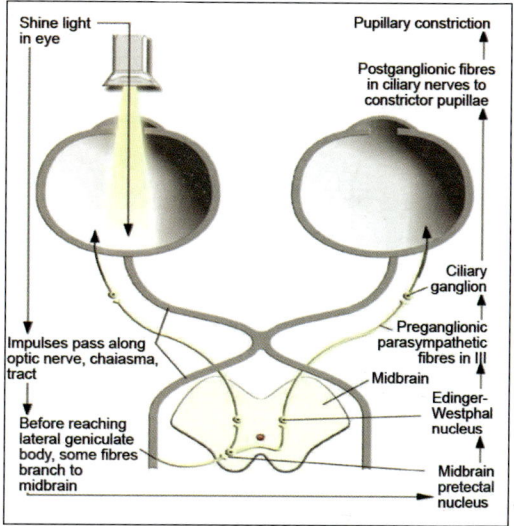

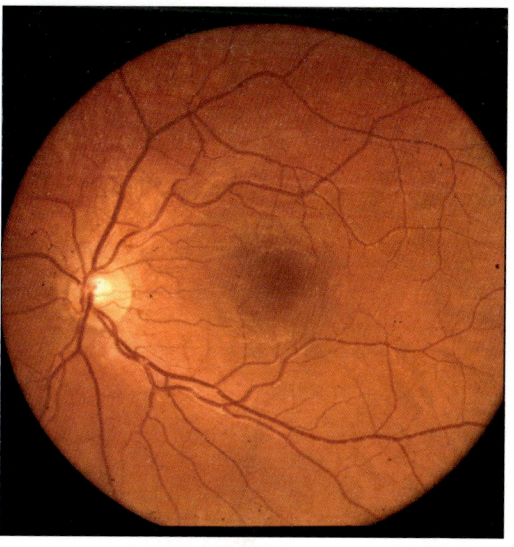

It is a part of routine physical or complete eye examination.

It is used to detect and evaluate symptoms of various retinal vascular diseases or eye diseases such as glaucoma.

It also indicated increased intracranial pressure which could be due to hydrocephalus or space occupying lesions in brain, etc.

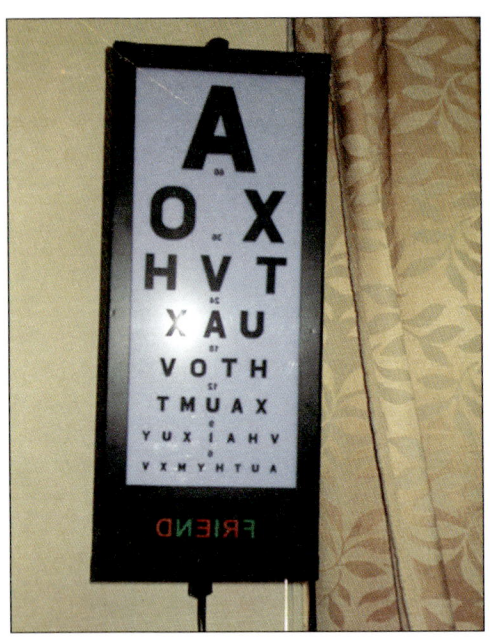
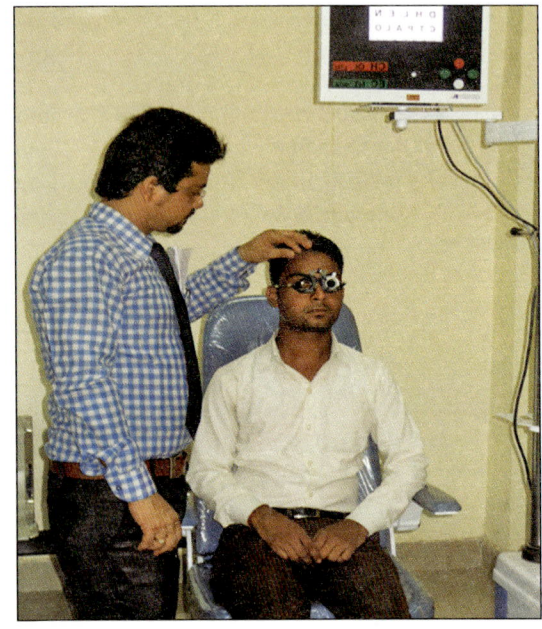

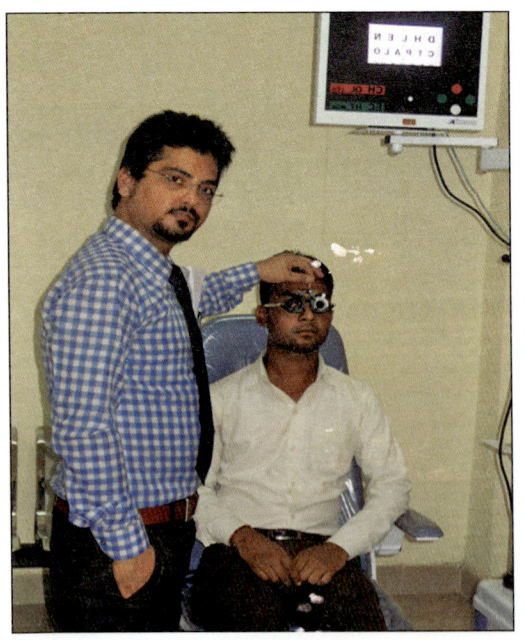
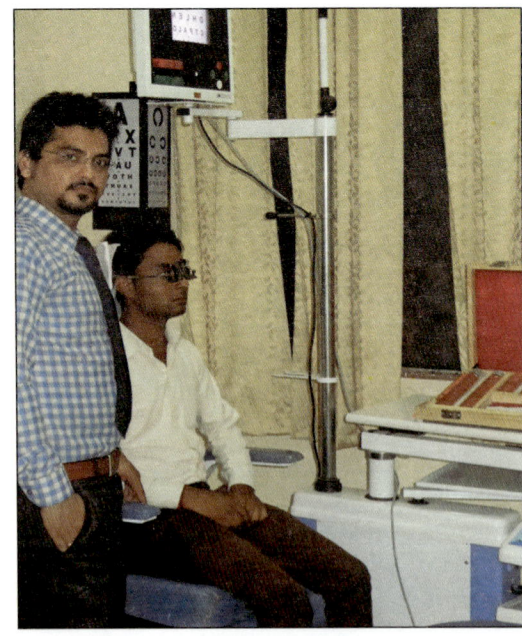

Superior rectus

Inferior oblique

Lateral rectus

Medial rectus

Inferior rectus

Superior oblique

Six cardinal direction movements of eyeball

OCULOMOTOR/TROCHLEAR AND ABDUCENS

a. The oculomotor, trochlear and abducens nerves are checked all together, as they are involved in eyeball movements supplying the extra ocular muscles.
b. These nerves allow smooth and coordinated movement in all directions of both eyes simultaneously.
c. Abducens supplies lateral rectus muscle and moves the eyeball down.
d. Trochlear supplies the superior oblique muscle and moves the eyeball down and rotates internally.
e. Oculomotor supplies all other muscles of eye movement and also helps in raising the eye lid and mediates pupillary constriction.

Procedure to test

- Ask the patient to keep the head immobile.
- Ask him/her to follow your finger with his/her eyes as you trace the letter "H".
- Alternatively, direct them to follow finger with their eyes as trace a large rectangle.
- Eyes should move in all diarections, in coordinated, smooth and symmetric fashion.

- Hold the eyes in lateral gaze for a few seconds to look out for nystagmus.

Trigeminal Nerve

The trigeminal nerve is involved in sensory supply to the face and motor supply to the muscles of mastication (temporalis and masseter).

There are 3 sensory branches of trigeminal nerve:

- Ophthalmic
- Maxillary
- Mandibular

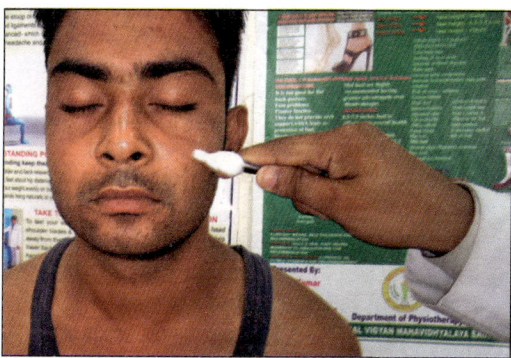

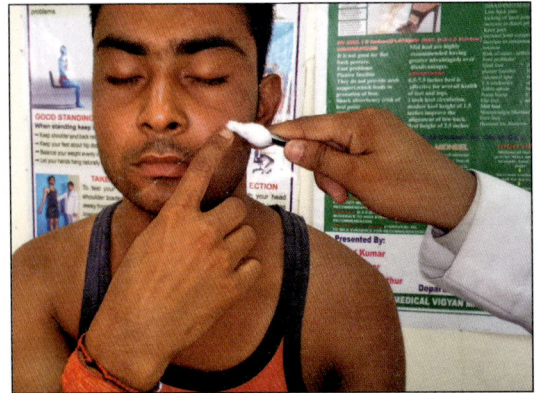

It also plays a role in the corneal reflex. Hence the trigeminal nerve is tested for:
1. Sensations over the face.
2. Motor and jaw jerk.
3. Corneal reflex sensory.

Sensations

- Ask the patient to close the eyes.
- Touch each of the 3 areas (ophthalmic, maxillary and mandibular).
- Around the jaw line, on the cheek and on the forehead lightly with the help of cotton.
- Later check with a pin for pain sensations.
- You can also check the temperature sensation, by using two test tubes of hot and cold water placed over these areas and ask the patient to identify the sensation.

Balint's syndrome: It is a triad of neuropsychological impairments, i.e. inability to perceive the visual field as a whole (Simultanagnosia), difficulty in fixating of eyes (Oculomotor apraxia) inability to move the hand to a specific object by using vision (optic ataxia).

Motor

- Ask the patient to clench the teeth together.

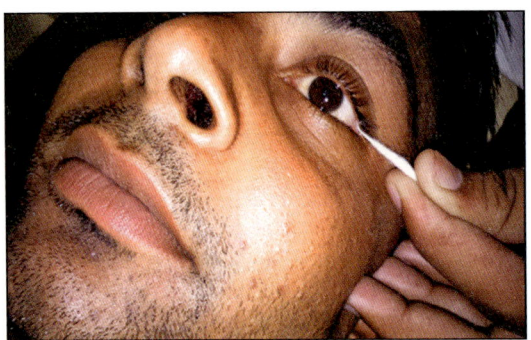

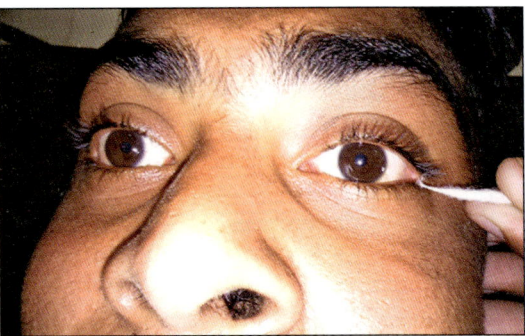

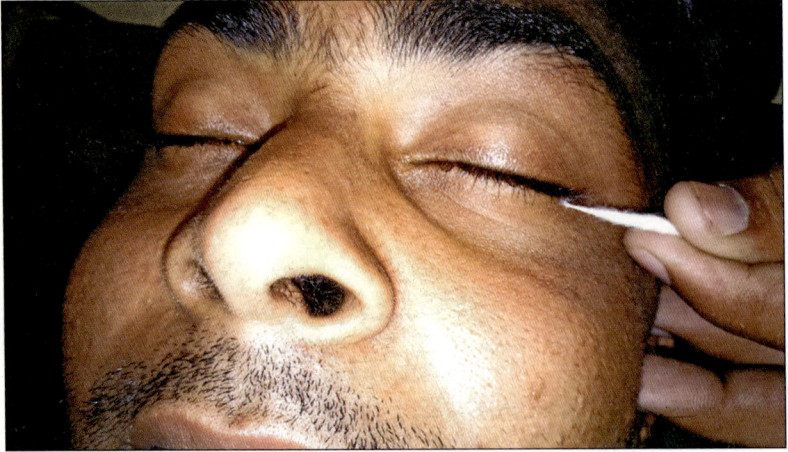

- Observe and palpate the bulk of the masseter and temporalis muscles.
- Now ask the patient to open the mouth and you resist it.

Jaw Jerk

- Place your non-dominant index finger on the patient chin.
- Strike your finger over the patient chin by a tendon hammer.
- The response is slight protrusion of the jaw.

Corneal Reflex

- Ask the patient to sit with open eyes and look straight.
- Lightly touch the cornea with a sterile cotton wool.
- The response will be shutting of the patient's eyelids.

Trigeminal neuralgia is also known as Prosopalgia characterized by episodes of intense pain in the face

FACIAL NERVE

The facial nerve is the 7th cranial nerve and supplies motor branches to the muscles of facial expression.

It also supplies anterior two-thirds of the tongue by its cauda tympanic branch which is sensory.

This nerve is tested by asking the patient to perform certain expressions on the face as follows:

- Make crease on the forehead.
- Close the eyes tightly.
- Puff out the cheeks.
- Smile by showing the teeth.

In UMN lesion of the facial nerve, there will be contralateral lower quadrant of the face affected and is termed as facial palsy.

In LMN lesion, there will be complete half of the face affected on the same side and is known as Bell's palsy.

VESTIBULOCOCHLEAR NERVE

It is the eighth cranial nerve and provides innervations to the hearing apparatus of the ear and also transmits information about balance and equilibrium to brain.

The vestibular and cochlear parts of this nerve are tested separately.

Cochlear part is involed in hearing, several tests are present to test this nerve.

Crude Tests of Hearing

Make the patient relax and rub your fingers next to either ear or wisper some words and ask the patient to repeat.

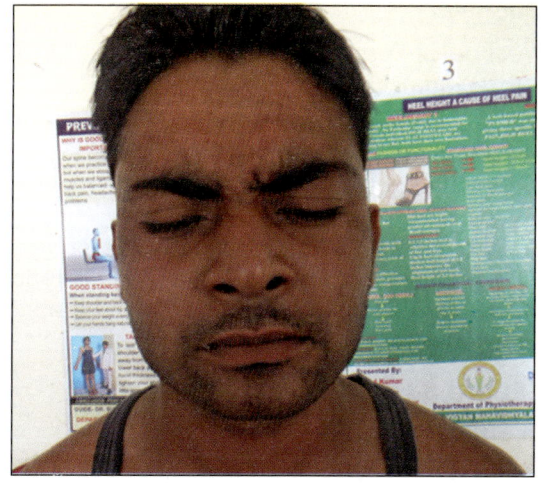
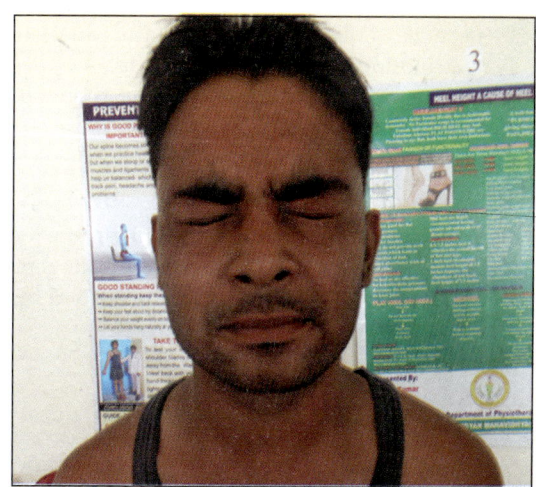

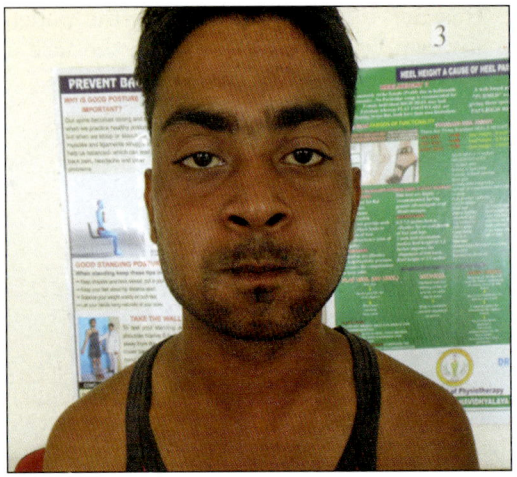 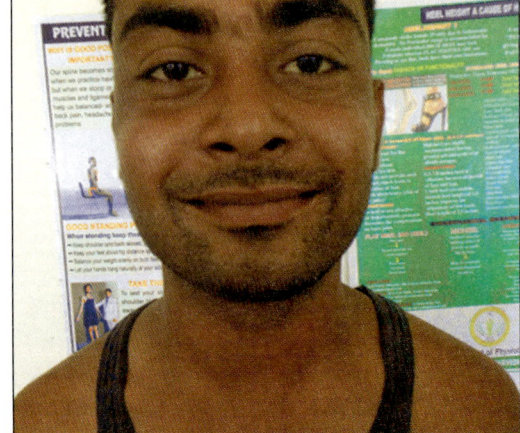

Weber Test

It is an easy screening test for hearing. This test is done to detect unilateral (oneside) conductive hearing and unilateral sensorineural hearing loss.

How to do?

For this test, a tuning fork of 512 Hz is used as it is within the range of normal hearing.
- Make the patient sit comfortably and explain him the entire procedure and take the consent.
- Get the tuning fork vibrate by striking ends against a rubber cork.
- Place vibrating fork on the midline of skull.
- The sound should be symmetrically heard on right and left ears equally.
- If there is conductive hearing loss (which may be because of obstructing wax in the canal), it is heard louder on the defective side.
- If there is sensorineural hearing loss, then it is heard louder on the normal side.

Rinne Test

The Rinne test is a hearing test and primarily used for testing the loss of hearing in one ear. It compares perception of sound transmitted by air conduction and by bone conduction

How to do?

- For this test, a 512 Hz tuning fork is used.
- Ask the patient to sit in relaxing position.

Explain the procedure to the patient and take consent.
- Get the tuning fork vibrate by striking ends against a rubber cork.
- Place the vibrating fork handle on the mastoid process behind the ear to be tested.
- Ask the patient to tell or raise hand when he stops hearing the sound.
- Once the hearing is stopped, place the tines of the fork next to the ear.
- In normal, the patient should hear the sound again as the air conduction is better than bone conduction.
- If the bone conduction is better than air conduction, this suggests a conductive hearing loss.
- If the airconduction is better than bone conduction, then it suggests a sensorineural hearing loss.

Vestibular Function

The vestibular apparatus of the inner ear is helpful to detect the movement of head and its position in space. If there is a damage to the vestibular system, then the chief symptom would be vertigo.

If the patient complains of vertigo, then DIX-Hallpike-test is done. It is a diagnostic maneuver used to identify benign paroxysmal positional vertigo (BPPV).

How to do ?

- Make the patient sit upright on the examination table with legs extended.

- The patient's head is then rotated to one side by 45 degrees.
- Then you assist the patient to lie down backwards quickly with the head held in approximately 20 degrees of extension.
- Now observe the patient's eye for about 45 seconds for onset of nystagmus, if there is a nystagmus, then the the test is positive.

GLOSSOPHARYNGEAL NERVE

It is the IX cranial nerve and is sensory for taste sensation supplying the posterior one-third of the tongue and palate. It is also involved in the gag reflex.

The glossopharyngeal nerve is best tested by checking the gag reflex.

How to do?

Touch the uvula with a tongue blade or a piece of cotton plug. The response will be reflex contraction of the back of the throat.

VAGUS NERVE

Vagus is the X cranial nerve. It provides motor supply to the pharynx. Vagal lesions produce palatal and pharyngeal paralysis, laryngeal paralysis and abnormalities of esophageal motility and other autonomic dysfunction.

How to Check?

- Listen to the patient talk as you are taking the history. A horeseness in the voice, whispering, nasal speech or the complaint of aspiration or regurgitation of foods, liquids through the nose is a striking feature of vagal lesions.
- Ask the patient to open the mouth and say "Ahh" as long as possible. You can use a tongue blade to depress the base of the tongue gently to observe.
- Observe the palatal arches as they contract and soft palate, in normal individuals, there is rise if palate and uvula is in central position and doesn't deviate.
- In vagal lesions, there is no elevation or constriction on the effected side.

SPINAL ACCESSORY NERVE

The spinal accessory nerve is the XI cranial nerve and gives motor supply to the sternocleido-mastoid and trapezius muscle. The main functions are:

- Rotation of the head to opposite side of the contrating muscle.
- Tilting of the head to the same side of the contracting muscle.
- Flexion of the neck by both sternocleidomas-toid muscle.
- Elevation of the shoulder.
- Drawing the head back such that the occiput tilts towards the acromion.

To check this nerve, the muscle power of the these two muscles is checked.

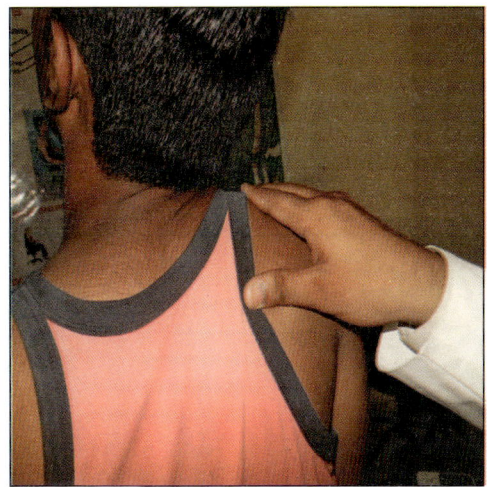

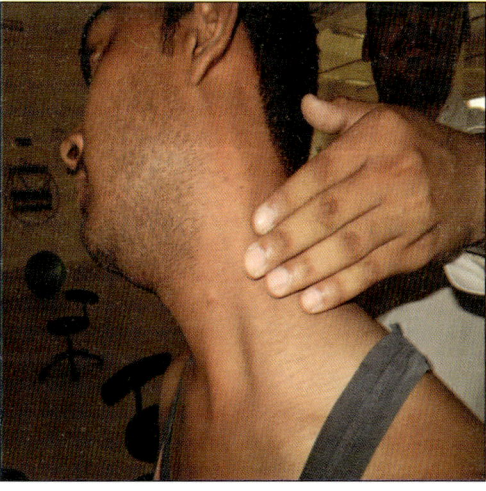

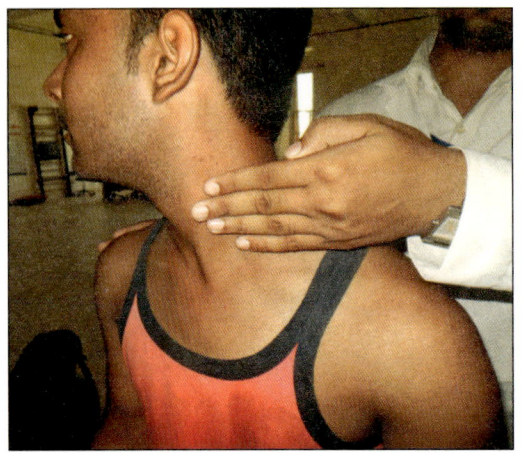
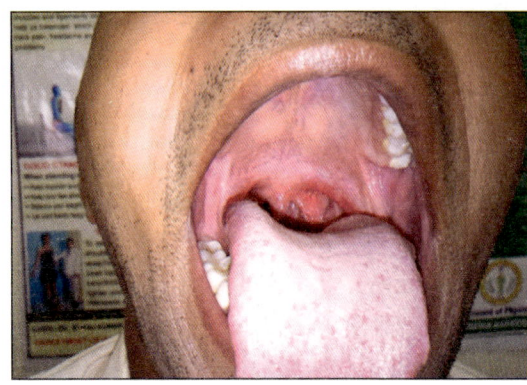

How to Check?

1. Palpate the trapezius and sternocleidomastoid muscle.
2. Ask the patient to perform the above mentioned movement first without resistance and later with resistance.
3. Compare the both sides.

Any weakness or paralysis of these muscles indicates the lesion of the nerve.

HYPOGLOSSAL NERVE

It is the XII cranial nerve and provides motor supply to the muscles of the tongue. The lesions of the hypoglossal nerve results in paralysis tand atrophy of the tongue muscles. There will be fasciculations of the tongue on the involved side.

How to Check?

Ask the patient to protrude the tongue out. Usually, in normal individuals, the tip of the tongue will be in center, if there is a lesion, the tip of the tongue will point to the normal side due to unopposed normal tone of unaffected side.

Also observe the tongue for atrophy and fasciculations.

8

Sensory Assessment

Superficial sensations:
a. Pain
b. Touch
- Fine
- Crude
c. Temperature

Deep sensations:
a. Pressure
b. Vibration
c. Joint position sense (proprioception)
d. Joint kinesthetic sense

Combined cortical sensation:
a. Tactile localization
b. Stereognosis (object recognition)
c. Two-point discrimination
d. Double simultaneous stimulation
e. Graphesthesia (traced figure identification)

Note. All assessment should be done with the patient's eyes closed after explaining the testing procedure to him.

SUPERFICIAL SENSATIONS

Pain

Test: Use safety pin or any object which is sharp enough to deflect the skin but not puncture it.

- Clean the instrument before administering the test and dispose it afterward.
- Apply sharp point to the patient's skin with a uniform pressure during each successive stimulus.
- Stimulus should not be applied too close to each other to avoid summation of impulses.

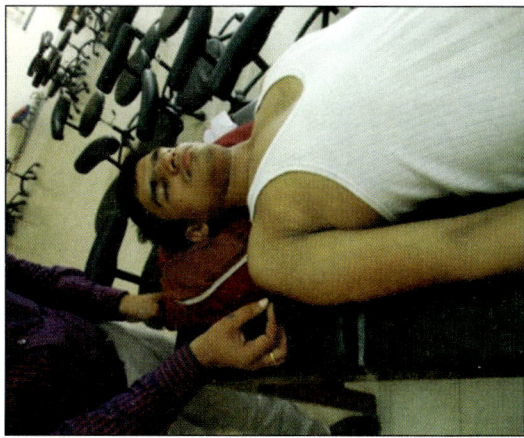

Response: Ask the patient to verbally indicate when a stimulus is felt.

Test all areas of the body.

Light Touch

Test: Use a camel hair brush or piece of cotton.

- Lightly touch or stroke the area to be tested.

Response: Ask the patient to indicate the stimulus by counting numbers.

- To avoid bias, trick the patient, by not giving the stimulus now and then.
- To find out the symmetry of sensation, compare with the normal and ask the patient to conform the symmetry of sensation.

Temperature

Test: Use two test tubes with stoppers.

- Fill one with warm water (40–45°C) and other with crushed ice (5–10°C).

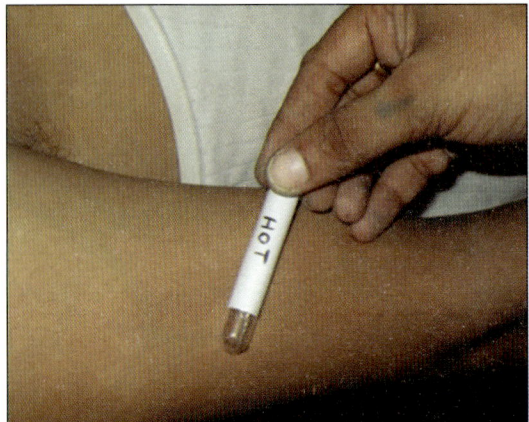 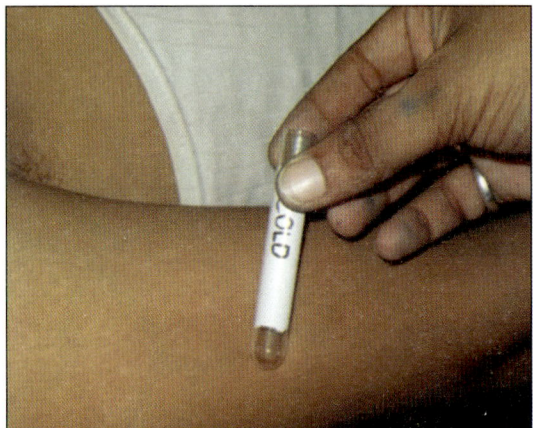

- Randomly place the test tubes over the skin area to be tested.

 Response: Ask the patient to indicate when a stimulus is felt by warm, cold or unable to tell.

- To avoid bias, trick the patient, by not giving the stimulus now and then.
- To find out the symmetry of sensation, compare with the normal and ask the patient to conform the symmetry of sensation.

DEEP SENSATIONS

a. Pressure

Test: Use your thumb or fingertip to apply a firm pressure on the skin surface.

 Response: Ask the patient to indicate the recognition of stimulus by saying yes or now.

- To avoid bias, trick the patient, by not giving the stimulus now and then.

- To find out the symmetry of sensation, compare with the normal and ask the patient to conform the symmetry of sensation.

b. Vibration

Test: A 128 Hz tuning fork is used.

- Randomly place the vibrating and non-vibrating tuning fork on a bony prominence.
- Use ear phones to avoid auditory clues.

 Response: Ask the patient to respond by saying vibrating or non-vibrating.

- To avoid bias, trick the patient, by not giving the stimulus now and then.
- To find out the symmetry of sensation, compare with the normal and ask the patient to conform the symmetry of sensation.

c. Joint Position Sense (Proprioception)

Test: Move the joint or extremity to be tested through an ROM and held in a static position.

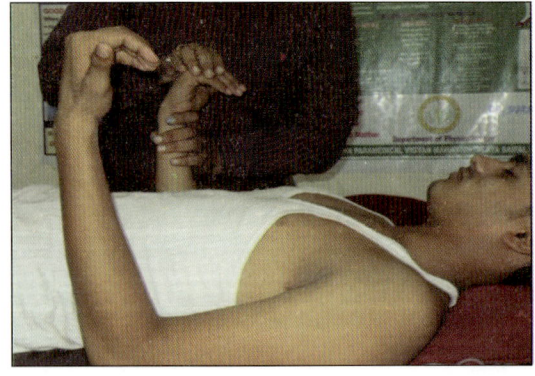 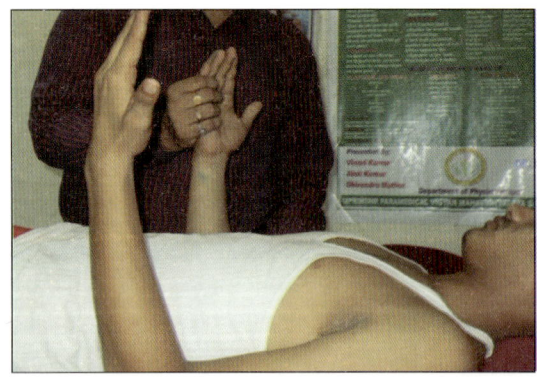

• Caution should be used with hand placements to avoid tactile stimulation.

Response: Ask the patient to describe the position of extremity verbally or to duplicate the position of extremity with contralateral extremity.

• To avoid bias, trick the patient, by not giving the stimulus now and then.
• To find out the symmetry of sensation, compare with the normal and ask the patient to conform the symmetry of sensation.

d. Joint Kinesthetic Sense (Awareness of Movement)

Test: Passively move the joint or extremity to be tested through a small range of motion.

Response: Ask the patient to indicate verbally the direction of movement while the limb is in motion or to duplicate simultaneously the movement with opposite limb.

• To avoid bias, trick the patient, by not giving the stimulus now and then.
• To find out the symmetry of sensation, compare with the normal and ask the patient to conform the symmetry of sensation.

COMBINED CORTICAL SENSATION

a. Tactile Localization

Test: Touch different skin surfaces of the patient with your fingertip.

Response: Ask the patient to identify the location of stimulus by pointing to the area or verbally.

Patient's eyes may be open during the response component.

• To avoid bias, trick the patient, by not giving the stimulus now and then.
• To find out the symmetry of sensation, compare with the normal and ask the patient to conform the symmetry of sensation.

b. Stereognosis (Object Recognition)

Test: Use familiar objects of different size and shape, e.g. keys, coins, pencil, comb, safety pin, etc.

Give a single object to the patient and ask him to identify it.

Response: Patient tells the name of that object.

Speech impaired patients select that particular item from a group after each test.

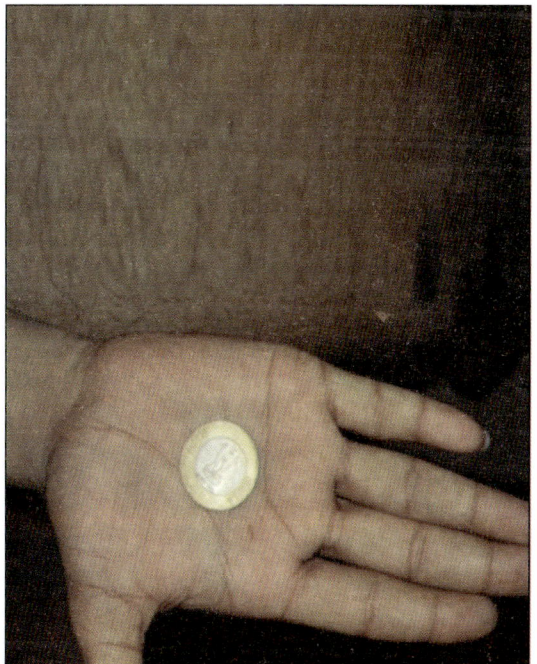
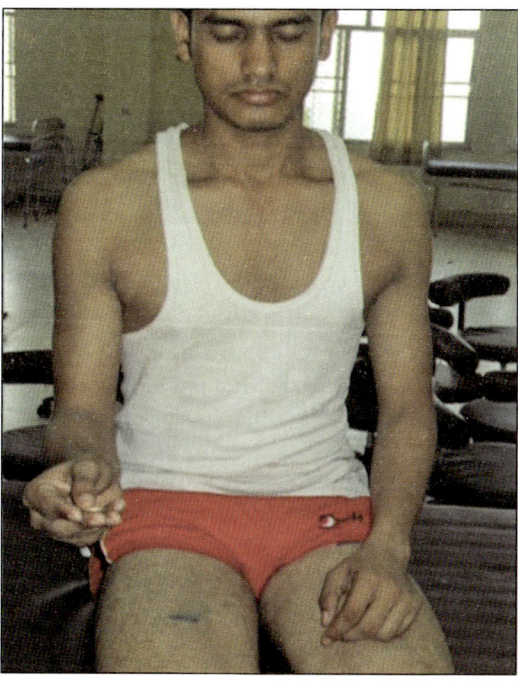

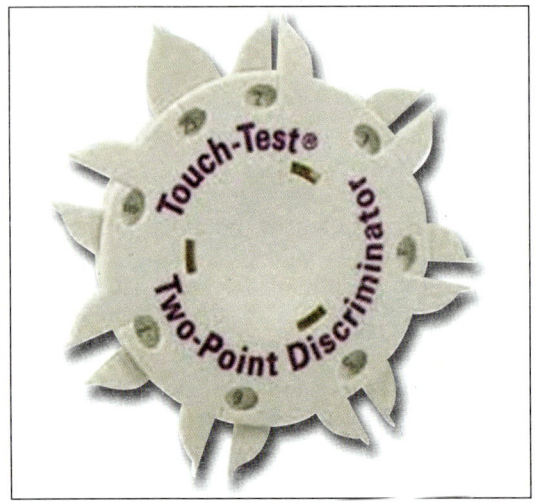

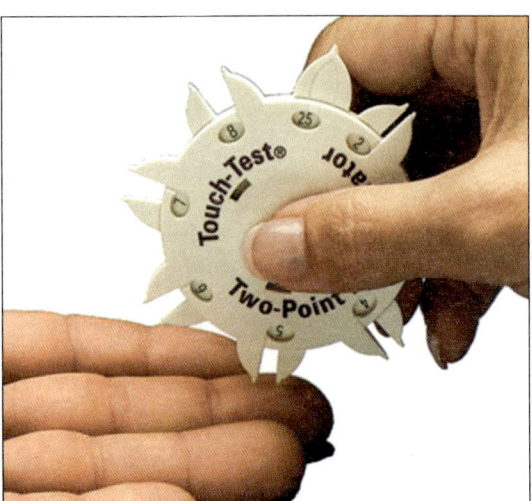

- To avoid bias, trick the patient, by not giving the stimulus now and then.
- To find out the symmetry of sensation, compare with the normal and ask the patient to conform the symmetry of sensation.

c. Two Point Discrimination

Test: It is a measure of the smallest distance between two stimuli (applied simultaneously and with equal pressure) that can still be perceived as two distinct stimuli.

- Use reshaped paper-clip with blunt ends or two-point discriminator.
- Apply the two tips of instrument to the patient's skin simultaneously.
- Gradually reduce the distance between two tips until the stimuli are perceived as one.
- Measure the smallest distance between the stimuli that is still perceived as two distinct points and record it.

Response: Ask the patient to identify the perception of 'one' or 'two' stimuli.

d. Double Simultaneous Stimulation

Test: It examines the ability to perceive a simultaneous touch stimulus on opposite sides of the body, proximally and distally on a single limb or proximally and distally on one side of the body.

Simultaneously, touch with finger-tip (with equal pressure)

- Identical locations on opposite side of the body.
- Proximally and distally on opposite side of the body.
- Proximal and distal locations on same side of the body.

Response: Ask the patient to verbally state when he or she perceives a touch stimulus and the number of stimuli felt.

e. Graphesthesia (Traced Figure Identification)

Test: It examines the ability to recognise the letters, numbers or designs traced on the skin by using the eraser end of a pencil.

- A series of letters, numbers or designs is traced on patient's palm.
- Gently wipe the palm with a soft cloth between each separate drawing.

Response: Ask the patient to identify verbally the figure drawn on the skin.

For patients with speech deficits select the figure from a series of line drawing.

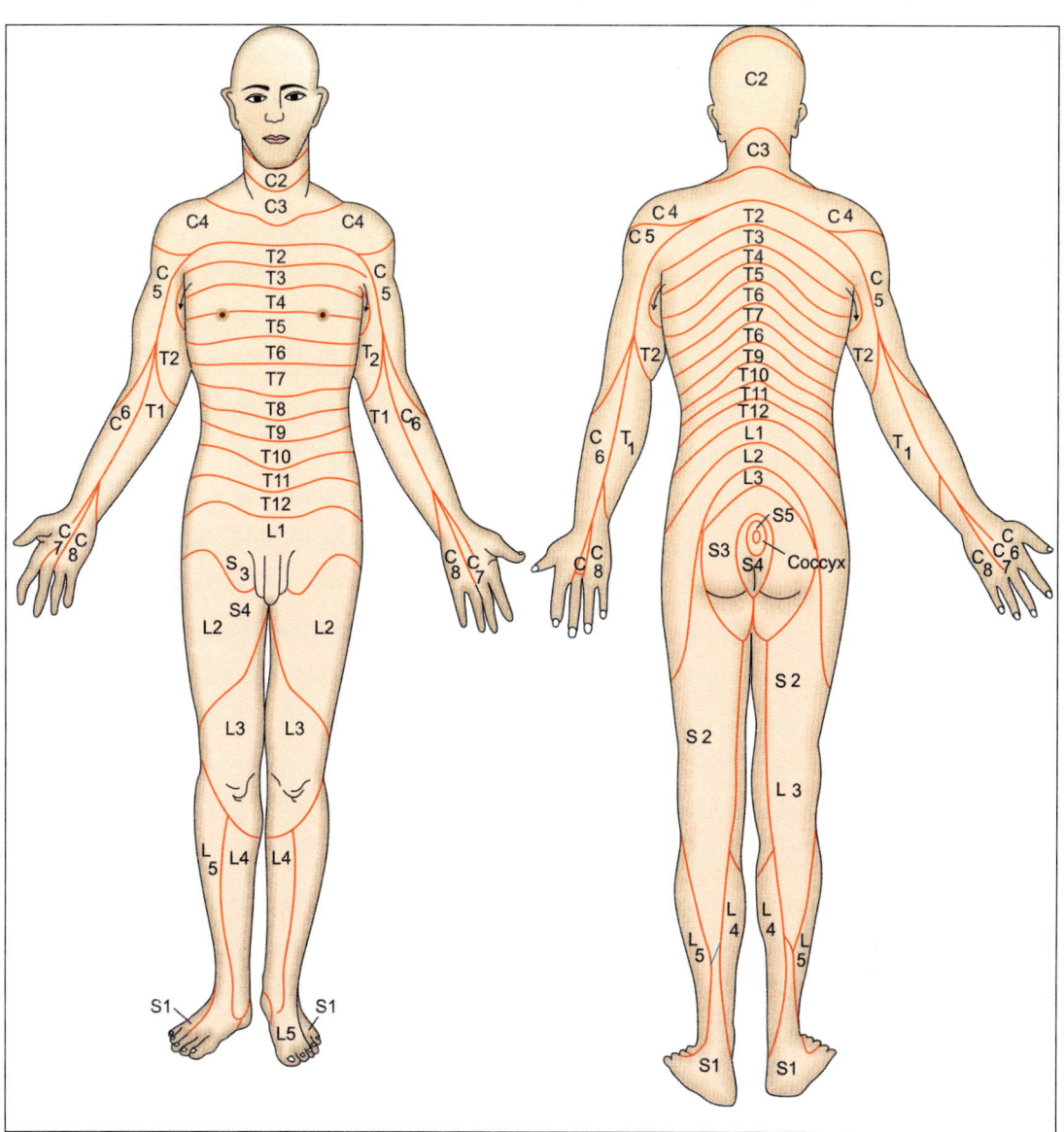

Body chart

9

Reflex Examination

A reflex is a stereotypic response to a stimulus.

Reflex testing helps to assess the relation and functions of both sensory and motor pathways and also connection between the peripheral nervous system and central nervous system.

Reflex testing helps us to identify the level of lesion in the nervous system.

It also helps to differentiate the UMN type of lesion to LMN type of lesion.

Clinically, the reflexes are classified into:

   a. Superficial
   b. Deep
   c. Pathological

In neurological diseases, normal physiological reflexes may be increased, decreased or lost and abnormal pathological reflexes may appear, especially with UMN lesion.

SUPERFICIAL REFLEXES

Most of the superficial reflexes are cutaneous reflexes where a tactile stimulus to a localized area of skin or mucous membrane results in a motor response except pupillary reflex where the pupil is stimulated by light. Some reflexes are cranial nerve-mediated and some spinal nerve-mediated.

Which reflexes do you need to check?

1. Pupillary reflex
2. Corneal reflex
3. Palpebral reflex
4. Gag reflex
5. Abdominal reflex
6. Cremastric reflex
7. Plantar reflex (Babinski sign) (it can be also noted as a pathological reflex)

Pupillary Reflex

- *Stimulus:* Light focused on the pupil.
- *Root value:* Cranial nerve II is afferent and III is efferent.
- *Response:* Constriction of pupil to light.

How to Check?

- Make sure that the room is dark and pupils are dilated a little.
- The room should not be completely dark that you can't observe the pupil reaction.
- Make the patient sit calmly on a chair and ask him to look straight.
- Now shine the light in right eye and observe the pupil being constricted.
- Now repeat the same procedure on left eye.

What do you Interpret?

- Usually the normal response of papillary reaction is described as "PERRLA" (pupils, equal, round, reactive to light accommodation).
- Abnormal responses are observed secondary to direct or indirect damage to optic nerve, parasympathetic injury or to the sympathetic neurons.
- Some sympathomimetics, like cocaine, will dilate the pupil and some narcotics, like heroin, will constrict the pupil.

Corneal Reflex

- *Stimulus*: Touching the cornea with a cotton plug.
- *Root value*: Cranial nerve V is afferent and VII is efferent.
- *Response*: Blinking of eyes.

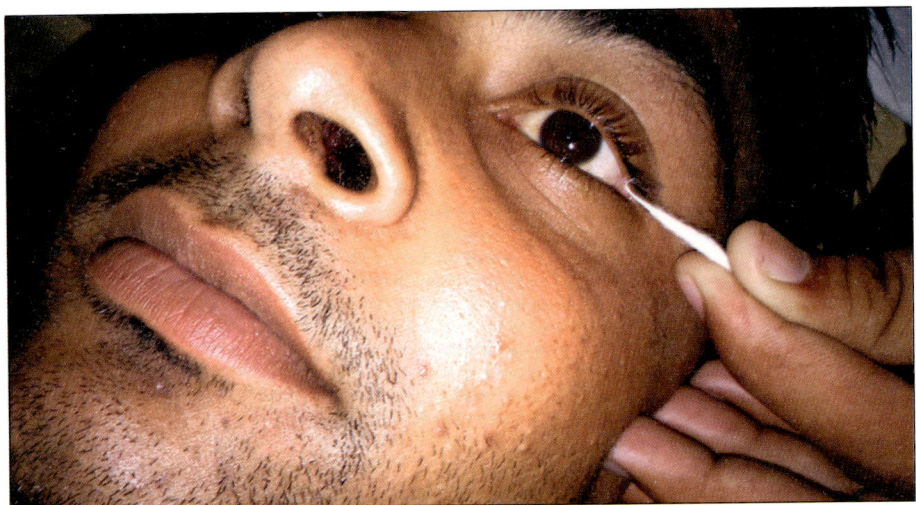

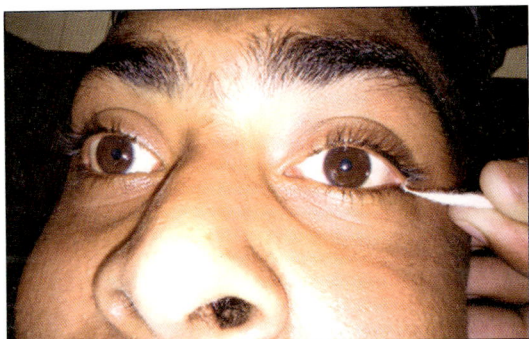
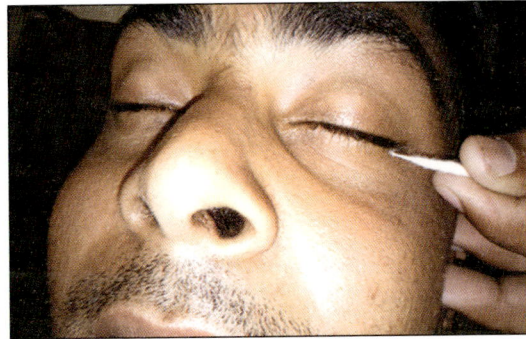

Before checking the corneal reflex, check whether your patient is wearing contact lens!!!

How to Check?

- Ask the patient to sit with open eyes and look straight.
- Lightly touch the cornea with a sterile cotton wool.
- The response will be shutting of the patient's eyelids.

What do you Interpret?

- An absent corneal reflex can be due to damage to trigeminal or facial nerve.
- It is also absent in facial muscle myopathy, Bell's palsy or brainstem disease.

- Chronic progressive external ophthalmoplegia.
- Contact lenses may diminish the reflex.
- In unconscious patient's, this reflex will indicate the functioning of the lower brainstem.
- You can't diagnose "brain dead" until the corneal reflex is absent.

Palpebral Reflex

- *Stimulus*: Touching the eyelids or eyelashes.
- *Root value*: Cranial nerve V is afferent and VII is efferent.
- *Response*: Blinking of the eyes.

How to Check?

- Ask the patient to sit with open eyes and look straight.

- Touch the eyelid or eyelash.
- The response will be shutting of the patient's eyelids.

What do you Interpret?

The reflex disappears in light to median plane of surgical anesthesia.

Gag Reflex

- *Stimulus*: Touching the soft palate around the tonsils area.
- *Root value*: Cranial nerve IX is afferent and X is efferent
- *Response*: Elevation of the palate and contraction of the muscle in the back of the throat (laryngeal spasm).

How to Check?

- Ask the patient to sit with mouth opened.
- Ask the patient to say "AAH".
- Touch the roof the mouth with a cotton bud.

In a study, it showed that 37% of healthy individuals don't have gag reflex.

Sword swallowers learn to suppress the gag reflex.

What do you Interpret?

In glossopharyngeal nerve palsy, the reflex is absent. Absence of gag reflex in stroke patients is an indication for dysphagia.

Abdominal Reflex

- *Stimulus*: Stroking over the skin on all quadrants of the abdomen around the umbilicus.
- *Root value*: T7 to T12 spinal segments.
- *Response*: Contraction of the abdominal muscles and retraction and deviation of the umbilicus towards the stimulus.

How to Check?

- Explain the entire procedure to your patient and take consent.
- Make the patient in supine lying.
- Expose the abdominal region in privacy.
- With the help of a blunt object (the tail-end of the reflex hammer will be beneficial), stroke firmly on the different quadrants of the abdomen.

Abdominal reflex is difficult to elicit in obese subjects and subjects with abdominal scars.

What do you Interpret?

- Abdominal reflex is reported as present/absent.
- An absent abdominal reflex can also a physiological response in obese patients, less tolerable patients, children, multiparous lax abdominal wall.
- It is pathological and can be due to neurological disturbances like spinal cord lesions involving

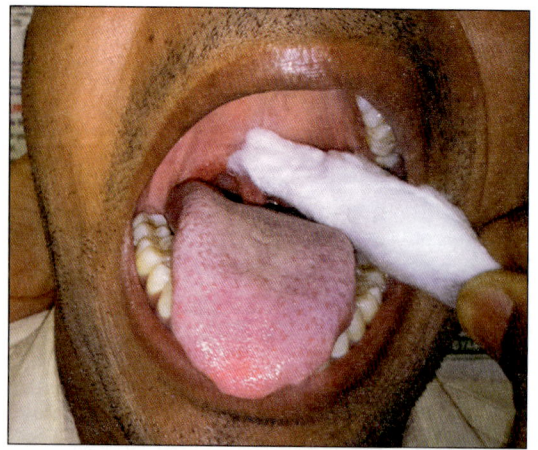

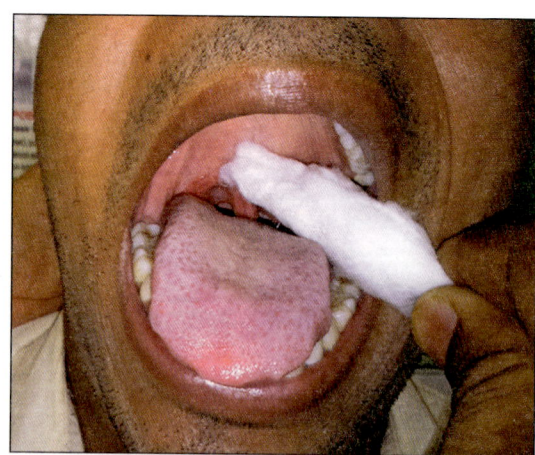

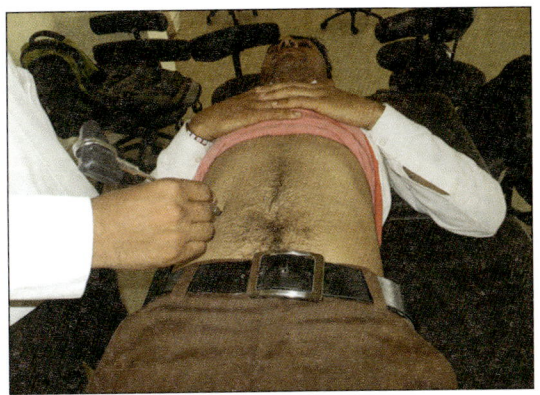 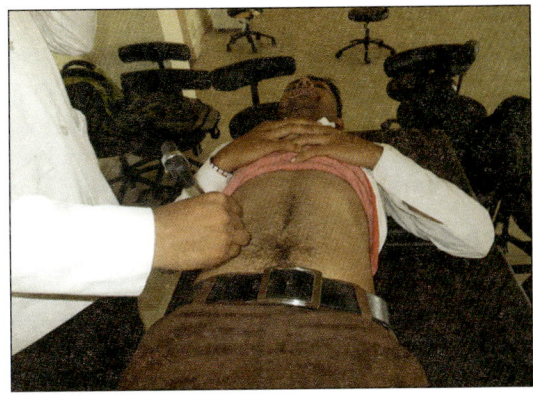

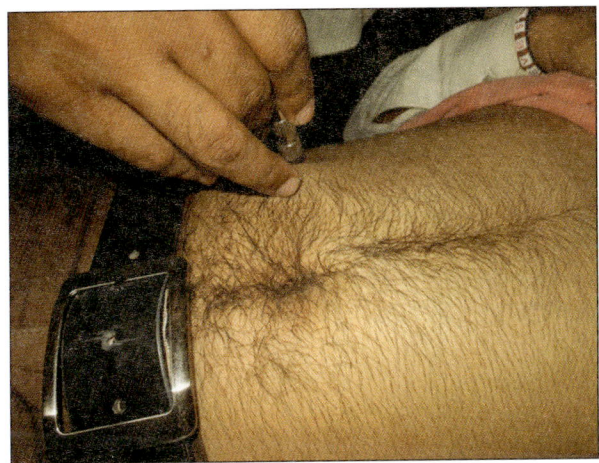

T7 to T12 segments, multiple sclerosis, motor neuron disease, etc.

Cremastric Reflex

- *Stimulus*: Stroking on the inner aspect of the thigh.
- *Root value*: L1 and L2 spinal segments.
- *Response*: Elevation of the ipsilateral testicle.

In boys, the cremastric reflex can be exaggerated which can occasionally lead to misdiagnosis of cryptorchidism.

How to Check?

- Explain the entire procedure to the patient and take consent.
- Have privacy settings, and make the patient lie supine with inner and upper part of the thigh exposed.
- Stroke in the inner and uppermost part of the thigh with a blunt object.

What do you Interpret?

- The reflex may be absent in the testicular torsion, LMN lesions and L1 L2 spinal cord injuries.
- In ilioinguinal nerve injuries the reflex is absent.
- It is a very helpful reflex for testicular emergencies.
- In genitofemoral nerve injuries, the reflex can be absent.

Plantar Reflex

Also known as Babinski reflex. It is a very reliable reflex to differentiate UMN and LMN lesion.

- *Stimulus*: Stroke the lateral aspect of the foot near heal. Apply steady pressure with the end of hammer towards the ball of the foot.
- *Root value*: L5 – S1
- *Response*: The response for the plantar reflex is described in the table below.

Babinski	Response	Interpretation/Result
Positive (+)	Extension of great toe with fanning of other toes	UMN lesion
Negative (-)	Flexion of the toes	Normal
Absent	No response is seen	LMN lesion.

DEEP REFLEXES

Deep tendon reflexes are also called as myotactic reflexes or muscle stretch reflexes.

They are elicited by the neurological hammer tap on a tendon which results in the brief or single contraction of the muscle.

What is the physiology behind?

When you tap the tendon of the muscle, it causes passive stretching of the muscle and neuromuscular spindles.

This activates sensory fibers which are afferent and results in the sufficient depolarization of the alpha motor neurons which are anterior horn cells at that level of the spinal segment.

The depolarization of motor nerve leads to the contraction of the muscle fibers which through the efferent nerve cause the muscle to contract.

What is a neurological hammer?

A neurological hammer which is also called as *percussion hammer* or *knee hammer* in some instances, which is an instrument used to assess the deep tendon relexes.

They come in different models.

Note: When you tap the tendon, immediately you should leave the touch of the hammer over the tendon to get a better response.

How you report the response?

Usually, in clinical scenario, the reflex response of the deep tendon reflexes are reported as follows based on the response.

Grade	Response
0	No response, reflex absent.
1	Decreased or diminshed response but response is present.
2	A normal response.
3	Exaggerated response or hyper-response.
4	Reflex elicitation results in clonus (Repetitive shortening of the muscle after a single stimulation).

What are the various deep tendon reflexes you check?

Reflex	Root value
Biceps jerk	C5,C6
Brachioradialis jerk	C5,C6
Triceps jerk	C7,C8
Knee jerk	L3,L4
Ankle/TA jerk	S1,S2

You can remember the root value of the reflexes by a rhyme you learned in your childhood:

1, 2 buckle my shoe (S1, S2—Ankle)

3, 4, kick the door (L3, L4—knee)

5, 6 pick up sticke (C5, C6—biceps)

7, 8 lay them straight (C7, C8—triceps)

Evaluation of reflexes at different levels of dysfunction of nervous system

Level of lesion	Response
Muscle	Stretch reflexes are depressed or lost.
Neuromuscular junction	Stretch reflexes are depressed or lost.
Peripheral nerve	Stretch reflex shows dimished or lost responses.
Nerve root	Stretch reflexes are depressed. Superficial reflexes are rarely depressed.
Spinal cord or brainstem	Stretch reflexes are diminished or lost at the level of lesion and exaggerated below the level of lesion.

Contd.

Contd.

	In stage of spinal shock, all reflexes below the level of lesion are diminished or lost. Superficial reflexes are diminished or lost at and below the level of lesion and above the level they show normal response.
Cerebellum	Stretch reflexes are hypoactive and pendular.
Basal ganglia	No change in the deep or superficial reflexes.
Cerebral cortex	Unilateral disease affecting the motor cortex will result in exaggerated responses in deep reflexes and absent abdominal and cremasteric reflexes on the contralateral side. The babinski is positive. Bilateral disease of cerebral cortex results in the same response as above, additionally primitive reflexes are seen.

Never tap directly over the cubital fossa, because it can cause rupture of the blood vessels in the fossa leading to hematoma.

Biceps Jerk

1. Explain the entire procedure to the patient.
2. Make the patient sit on a chair or attain a supine lying if patient can't sit.
3. Support the patient forearm in flexed elbow at 90 degrees in mid pronated forearm.
4. Palpate the tendon of biceps in the cubital fossa and place your thumb in it.
5. Now tap on your thumb.

Response: Flexion of the elbow.

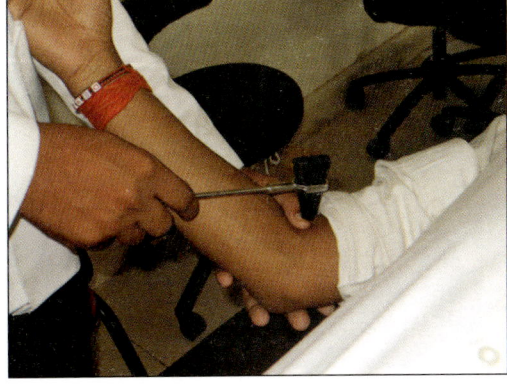

Checking the biceps jerk

Brachioradialis Jerk

1. Explain the entire procedure to the patient.
2. Make the patient sit on a chair.
3. Support the patient forearm in flexed elbow at 90 degrees in mid-pronated forearm.
4. As the tendon is not so easily palpated, so tap on the forearm just approximately 10 cm proximal to wrist.

Response: A normal response is flexion of the arm at elbow with supination.

Triceps Jerk

1. Explain the entire procedure to the patient.
2. Make the patient to sit or attain a supine lying position, if the patient can't sit.

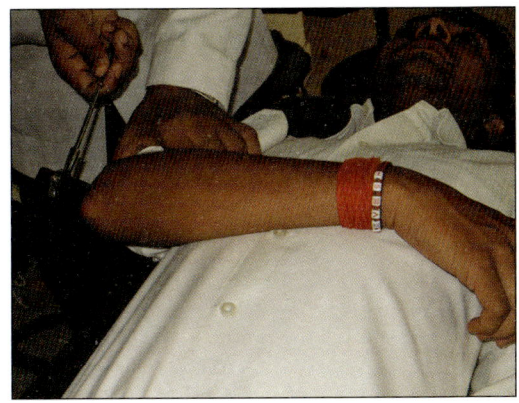

Triceps jerk

3. In sitting position, pull the patient arm off the body such that the arm forms a rough right angle at the shoulder. Flex the elbow.
4. Now feel the triceps tendon as a broad structure above the olecranon process.
5. Now tap on the tendon of the triceps and observe the response.
6. If the patient is lying, just make the patient arm adducted and flex the elbow to 90 degrees such that the forearm rests on the abdomen of the patient.
7. Now feel the tendon of the triceps and tap.

Response: There will be extension of the forearm.

Knee Jerk/Quadriceps Jerk

1. Explain the entire procedure to the patient.
2. Make the patient sitting on a high chair, feet off the ground or make the patient lie supine on the examination couch.

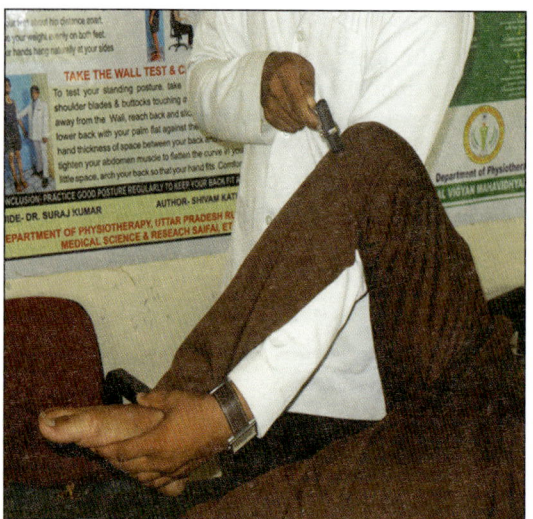
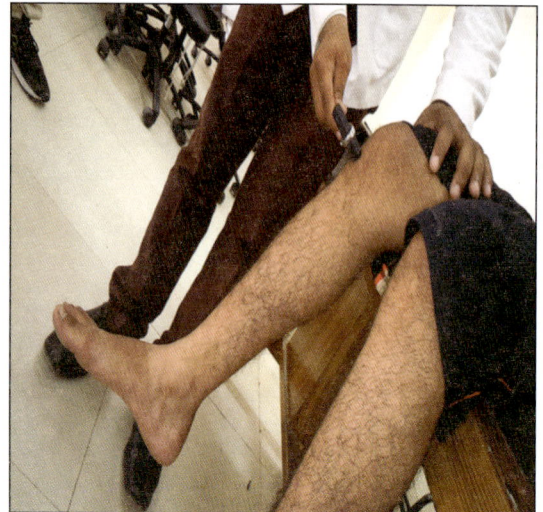

Knee jerk

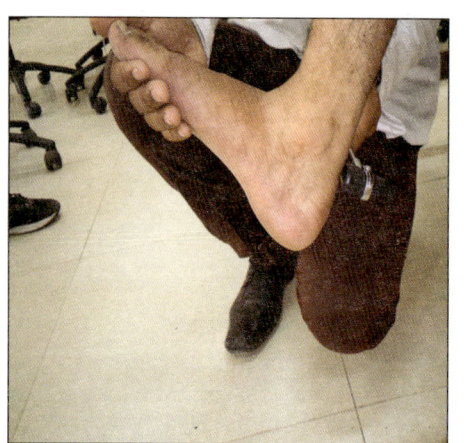
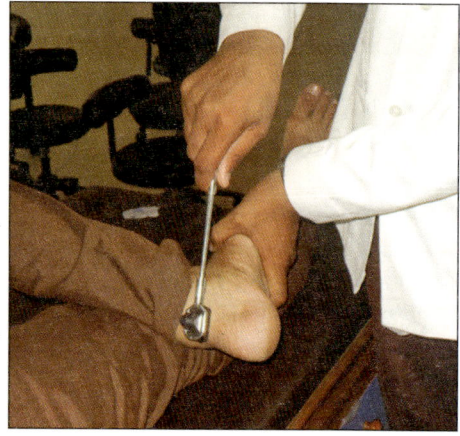

TA jerk

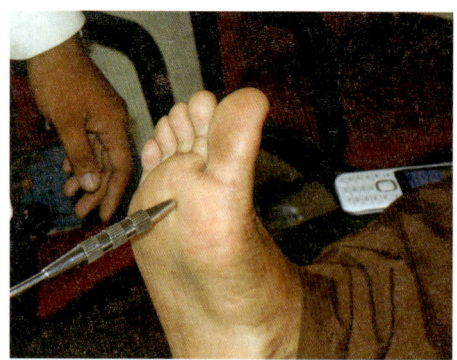
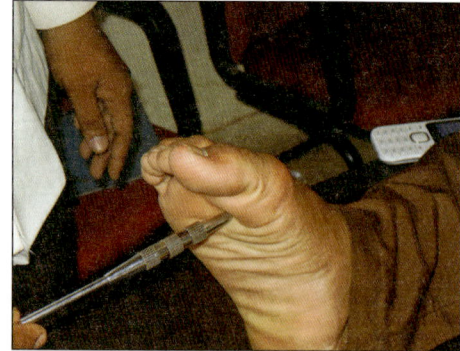

Plantar reflex

3. In sitting position, palpate the tendon of the quadriceps just below the patella.

4. Now tap directly over the tendon and observe the response.

5. In lying position, flex the knee, by placing your fist or a roll of towel under the knee so that the knee is flexed.

6. Now feel the tendon and strike.

Response: In normal response, there will be extension of the knee.

Ankle Jerk/TA Jerk

1. Explain the entire procedure to the patient.

2. Make the patient sitting on a high chair, feet off the ground or make the patient lie supine on the examination couch.

3. In sitting position, dorsiflex the foot so that it makes a right angle with the lower leg.

Now tap on the tendon above the calcaneum on the posterior part of the leg.

Response: Plantar flexion of the foot.

Important Points to Note

1. In sensory neuron disorders, like diabetic polyneuropathies, there will be delay in the transmission of impulse to the reflex center (spinal cord), hence there will be diminished or lost responses observed.

2. In peripheral motor neuropathies, which are LMN lesions, there will be lost or diminished reflexes because of disorder in the motor neuron.

3. In a disease of the neuromuscular junction or myopathies (muscle disorders), there will be loss of reflexes.

4. Some diseases which are systemic, like thyroid disorders, may have their impact on the reflexes, e.g. in hyperthyroidism, the reflexes will be exaggerated.

10

Motor Examination

In motor examination, we examine not only the affected muscle strength but also coordination, ranges, muscle atrophy, assessment of muscle tone (e.g. clasp knife spasticity or lead pipe rigidity), disturbances of the movements, muscle endurance (fatigability), any spontaneous movements in the form of fasciculations or twitches, muscle tightness, any asymmetry or deformity, etc.

TONE

The tension within the muscle in relaxed position.
• It is checked for normal/hypotonicity/hypertonicity.
• Preparation of the patient:
    1. Patient should be comfortable.
    2. Relaxed
    3. Cooperative.

Procedure

a. Place your hands under patient hand/wrist/elbow or place to be tested one hand will initiate the movement passively and other will stabilize.
b. Check for resistance whether it is increased or decreased.

Testing of Tone

1. It is tested by fast passive movements.
2. Note the degree of resistance/tension/extensibility/range after passive stretching.
3. It must be graded as mild/moderate/severe.

Increase in Tone

1. Spasticity
    a. *Clasp knife*: Initial resistance terminal free to move (upper motor neuron lesion).
2. Rigidity
    a. *Cog wheel*: A steady increase in resistance throughout the movement (extra-pyramidal lesion).
    b. *Lead pipe*: An increase in resistance throughout the movement (extra-pyramidal lesion).

Decrease in Tone

1. *Floppy baby syndrome*: Infantile hypotonia (generalised decrease in muscle tone).
2. *Impaired muscle tone*: Akinetic epilepsy (drop attack or drop seizure) or cataplexy (tone is decreased after strong emotions, e.g. laughing, etc.

3. *Babinski tonus test*

Patient position	Procedure	Normal response	Abnormal response	Diagnosis
Supine/sitting	Arms are abducted and elbow is passively flexed	Tone maintained; Easily done.	Increase flexibility	Hypotonicity
			Reduce flexibility	Hypertonicity

4. *Head dropping test*

Patient position	Procedure	Normal response	Abnormal response	Diagnosis
Supine and re-laxed; attention diverted	Lifts patient head with right hand and allow it to drop on left palm of therapist	Head drops suddenly	Head drops slowly, gently, etc.	Extrapyramidal lesion

5. *Shoulder shaking test*

Patient position	Procedure	Normal response	Abnormal response	Diagnosis
Supine/ sitting	Shake the patient shoulder briskly back and forth	Reciprocal motion of the arm	Decreased arm swinging Greater arm swinging	Extrapyramidal lesion Cerebellar diseases

6. *Arm dropping test*

Patient position	Procedure	Normal response	Abnormal response	Diagnosis
Supine/sitting	Patients arm raised briskly to shoulder level and then dropped	Arm drops suddenly	Arm drops slowly	Spasticity
			Arms drop more rapidly than normal	Flacidity

- If tension is increased in muscles it is necessary to find out whether it is due to muscle level (stiffness) or neurological level.
- Presence of tone increased to passive movements should be graded under modified Ashworth scale (MAS).

- Many cases like hemiplegia, cerebral palsy, etc. make the movement difficult and sometimes impossible and these kinds of movement can be graded under voluntary motor control.

Modified Ashworth Scale (MAS)

Grades	Description
0	No increase in muscle tone.
1	Slight increase in muscle tone with catch and release at the end.
1+	Slight more increased range as catch and followed by release for half of the range.
2	Resistance is increased throughout the range during passive movements but part moved freely.
3	Passive movements difficult with considerable increased muscle tone.
4	Part remain rigid in flexion or extension.

VOLUNTARY CONTROL TESTING

- These grades are used during examination procedures.

Grades of voluntary motor control testing

Grades	Description
1+	Gravity eliminated plane with 1/3rd movement possible.
1++	Gravity eliminated plane with 2/3rd movement possible.
1+++	Gravity eliminated plane with full range of motion.
2+	1/3rd movement possible against gravity.
2++	2/3rd movement possible against gravity.
2+++	Full range possible against resistance.
3+	1/3rd movement possible against gravity.
3++	2/3rd movent possible against gravity.
3+++	Full range possible against gravity.
4	Skilled movements.

Synergy

- It is an abnormal stereotyped primitive mass movement pattern associated with spasticity and which can be triggered either reflexively or voluntarily.
- It can be either flexor synergy or extensor synergy.
- It involves the action of certain muscles in combination that produces abnormal pattern which are not useful for functional activities.

Abnormal synergy in upper and lower limbs

Flexion synergy for upper limbs	Flexion synergy for lower limbs	Extension synergy for upper limbs	Extension synergy for lower limbs
Shoulder girdle retraction and elevation, shoulder abduction, external rotation, supination, flexion of elbow, wrist and finger flexion.	Hip flexion, abduction and lateral rotation, knee felxion, dorsiflexion and inversion.	Shoulder girdle protraction and depression, shoulder adduction, internal rotation, elbow extension, pronation, wrist and finger flexion.	Hip extension, adduction, internal rotation, knee extension, ankle plantar flexion, inversion, and plantar flexion.

Muscle that do not take part in either of the synergies are:

1. Latissmus dorsi
2. Teres major
3. Serratus anterior
4. Wrist and finger extensors
5. Ankle evertors

Synergies are different from the abnormal attitude seen in a hemiparesis patient. The abnormal hemiplegic attitude is due to the combination of strongest component of the flexor and extensor synergy in both upper and lower limbs.

Grades of Voluntary Control Testing
(For assessing synergy pattern)

Grades	Description
0	No contraction.
1	Initiation of contraction or flicker contraction.
2	Half range of motion in pattern.
3	Full range of motion in pattern.
4	Initial half range in isolation and the later half in pattern.
5	Full range of motion in isolation but goes into pattern when resistance offered.
6	Full range of motion in isolation against resistance.

Muscle Tightness

- It should be checked for upper limb as well as lower limbs.

- The tightness is more commonly seen in biarticular muscles, e.g. hamstring, biceps, TA, rectus femoris, etc.
- It is necessary to find out the muscles that develop contractures.

Clonus (steps to follow)

- Patient must be relaxed.
- Apply sudden sustained flexion to ankle.

Response: Few oscillatory beats in normal subject but if persist it causes increase tone.

Range of Motion (Power)

- A patient cooperation is needed.
- These are active procedures and these cannot be done in unconscious patients, infants, mentally retarded patients, etc.
- Isometric manual muscle testing procedure is performed in case of muscle weakness or where there is difficulty in initiating the movements.
- In such conditions, select muscle to be tested to avoid tricks movements.
- Stabilize the proximal joint so that prime movers can move freely, e.g. fix the arm distally so that the forearm can move freely for pronation in case of muscle weakness, etc.
- Ask the patient to hold the arm outstretched for up to 1 minute in supination with eyes closed, the weak arm will gradually pronates and drift downwards.

Testing few muscles of upper extremity and lower extremity

	Root value	Muscle	Nerve	Action	Response
1	C5, C6 and C7	Serratus anterior	Long thoracic nerve	Press arm against wall	Look for winging of scapula
2	C6, C7 and C8	Tricep	Radial nerve	Elbow extension	Arm will extend against resistance
3	L1, L2, L3	Illiopsoas	Femoral nerve	Hip flexion	Hip will flexed against resistance
4	L5, S1 and S2	Gluteus maximus	Inferior gluteal nerve	Hip extension	Patient attempt to keep heel on the bed against resistance
5	L5, S1 and S2	Hamstring	Sciatic nerve	Knee flexion	Pulling of heel towards buttocks against resistance to maintain this position
6	S1 and S2	Gastrocnemeus, soleus	Tibial nerve	Plantar flexion	Maintaining ankle plantar flexion against resistance

Manual muscle testing (MMT) grades

Grade	Description
0	No contraction.
1	Flicker of contraction.
2	Full range of motion in gravity eliminated plane.
3	Full range of motion against gravity.
4	Full range of motion against gravity and against half of maximal resistance.
5	Full range of motion against gravity and against maximal of resistance.

11

Gait Assessment

PARAMETERS OF GAIT

1. **Pelvic rotation**
   - The pelvis rotates by 4° on either side during walking.
   - By this, excursion of COG reduces and elevates COG by 6/16″.
2. **Pelvic tilt:** Pelvis drops on the side of swinging leg during walking to save the vertical rise of COG by 3/16″.
3. **Knee flexion:** The knee bends minimally on the stance leg during mid-stance, which decreases its length and also the height of COG by 7/16″.
   Total saving in vertical excursion of COG is 7/16′ + 6/16″+3/16″= 1 inch.
4. **Knee and ankle movement:** Movements occur between knee, ankle, subtalar and mid-tarsal joints to smoothen the amplitude of COG to 2″ by flexing, extending, pronating and supinating these joints in a coordinated manner.
5. **Pelvic sway:** Sideways sway of pelvis brings the COG over one leg during stance and produces a side to side sinusoidal curve.
6. **Limb rotation:** The leg internally rotates 25 degrees on stance and externally rotates on swing to smoothen the sideways curve of COG.
7. **Stride length:** Linear distance between two successive phases of the same foot.
8. **Step length:** Distance between heel strike of one foot and heel strike of other foot (1/2 of stride length).
9. **Stride width:** Distance between midline of one foot and midline of other foot.
10. **Toe out angle:** Angle made by midline of foot to direction of propulsion (6–7°).
11. **Cadence:** Number of steps per unit time generally minutes (60–120 steps per minute).

GAIT ANALYSIS

Ask the patient to walk and observe his walking pattern carefully for following findings/points: Gait is symmetrical or asymmetrical?

- If symmetrical, look for conditions shown in Flow chart 1.
- If asymmetrical, look for conditions shown in Flow chart 2.

PATHOLOGICAL GAITS

Any deviations from the normal gait pattern are considered to be abnormal or pathological gaits. Some of the pathological gaits which are encountered by the physiotherapist in his routine practise are discussed below.

1. **Antalgic gait:** It is also known as painful gait. It is self-protective and may be seen in injuries to pelvis, hip, knee, ankle or foot. In this gait, the patient tries to remove weight on the affected limb as early as possible. As a result, the stance phase of affected limb is shorter than unaffected side.
2. **Athrogenic gait:** The athrogenic gait is because of stiffness or deformity at pelvis, hip joint, knee joint or ankle. It may be painful or painless. The patient with this gait usually lifts entire lower limb higher than normal to clear the ground because of joint stiffness. When the affected is bearing weight, the gait length is smaller.

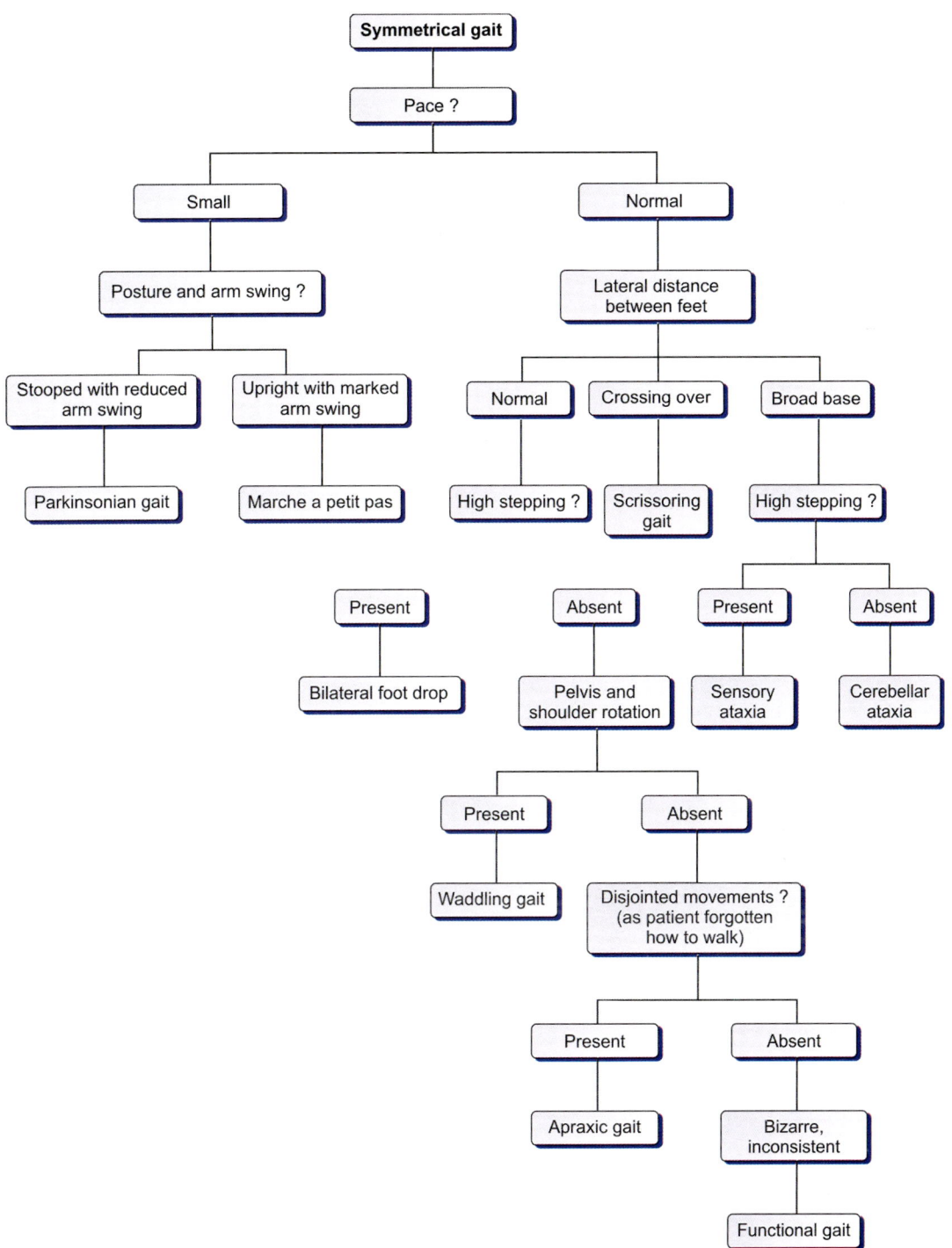

Flow Chart 1

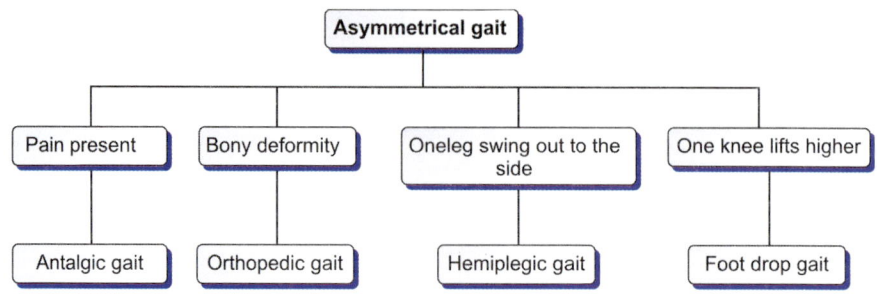

Flow Chart 2

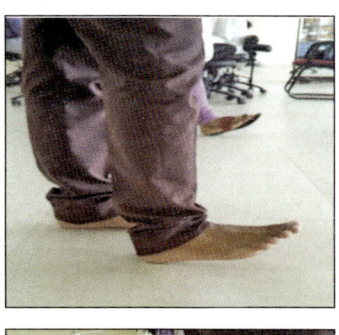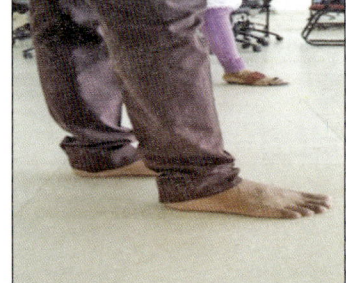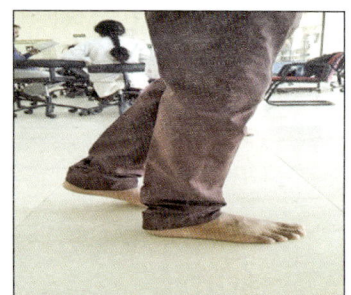

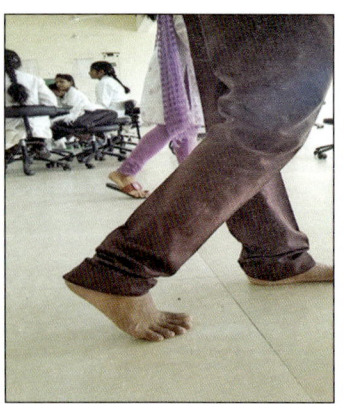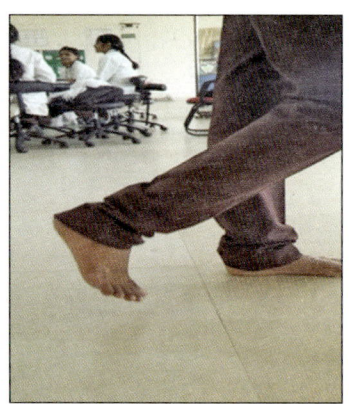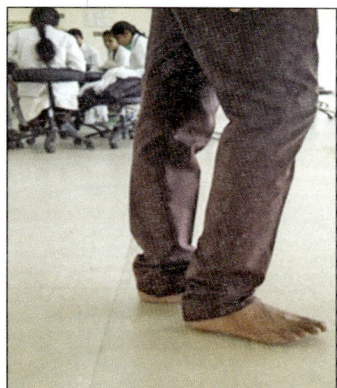

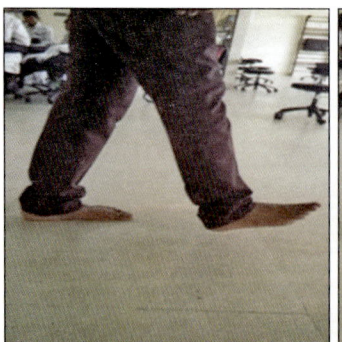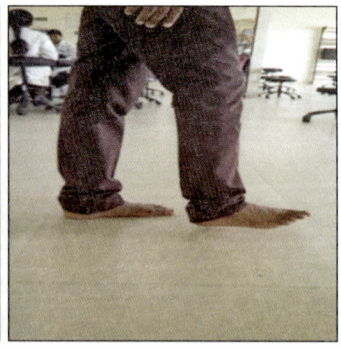

3. **Ataxic gait:** It is because of incordination and poor balance. It is characterized by wide base of support. The gait is irregular, jerky and weaving.

4. **Trendelenburg's gait:** It is due to weakness or paralysis of hip abductor muscles. The patient exhibits excessive lateral flexion of spine inorder to compensate the pelvic drop. If there is weakness of abductors bilaterally, then the patient shows "wobbing" or "chorusgirl swing" gait.

5. **Equinus gait:** This gait is seen in talipes equinovarus. Weight of the body falls on dorsolateral edge of foot.

6. **Hemiplegic gait:** The patients with hemiplegia (paralysis of one-half of body) swing the affected lower limb in a circle. In addition, the affected upper limb is carried across the trunk for balance.

7. **Parkinsonian gait:** It is also called as festinating gait. It is seen in patients suffering from parkinsonism. It is characterized by short rapid steps. The arms are held stiffly and do not have associate movement. The patient may lean forward and walk.

8. **Hand to knee gait:** It is seen in patients whose quadriceps muscle is injured or paralysed. This type of gait is usually seen in poliopatients. The patient pushes back the knee into hyperextension with hand in order to compensate.

9. **Scissoring gait:** This type of gait is due to spasticity (increased tone) of hip adductor muscles which causes the knees to be drawn together. This type of gait is seen in spastic paraplegics and cerebral palsy kids.

10. **Short leg gait:** If one leg is shorter than the other, the patient demonstrates a lateral shift to the affected side. The patient may evert the foot on the affected side trying to "lengthen" the limb.

12

Bladder and Bowel Assessment

The bladder and bowel assessment is very important aspect in neurological assessment to identify the neurogenic bladder.

A neurogenic bladder is a dysfunction of urinary bladder, where a patient loses his control over the bladder due to disease or damage/injury to the brain, spinal cord or nerves.

UMN NEUROGENIC BLADDER

Also known as spastic bladder or reflex bladder. Spinal cord injuries that occur above conus medullaris leave the S2–S4 levels of the spinal cord segments leaving them intact. This means that all the spinal and autonomic nerves located in these level can still be functional in a reflex way (unconscious way).

The detrusor muscles are likely to signal your brain with only smaller amount of urine because of this.

There is a detrusor muscle dyssynergia meaning the timing between bladder muscle and the external sphincter contract at the same time leading to development of outpouchings of the bladder wall and reflux of urine into the ureters and kidneys.

LMN NEUROGENIC BLADDER

Also known as flaccid bladder. Spinal cord injuries that occur at or below the conus medullaris damage the nerves that are involved with the bladder function. In these injuries, there is no reflex nerve activity and the bladder no longer functions and is in flaccid state.

There will be incontinence due to loss of tone in the external sphincter.

HOW TO ASSESS THE PATIENT?

- The assessment of the patient with bladder and bowel dysfunction starts with the taking consent from the patient.
- Take a clear history that include medical and surgical history, history of medications used or being used, history of neurological dysfunction, OBG history.
- You may need to ask the following questions:
  - How many days are you suffering from the symptoms?
  - What are the aggrevating factors?
  - What is the frequency of the passing urine in 24 hrs?
  - Do you need to rush to the toilet?
  - When you pass the urine, is it coming continuously or interrupted?
  - Do you get the feeling that you have completely emptied the urine?
  - Do you ever leak when you cough, sneeze, laugh or jump?
  - Do you have a history of urinary tract infection in the past 6 months or a regular history of UTI?

After that, check the patient's bowel habits.

A fluid input/output chart can be reviewed from the nurses notes.

A bladder and bowel scan can be helpful in identifying the problem.

13

ADL Assessment

ACTIVITIES OF DAILY LIVING ASSESSMENT

The physiotherapist's ultimate aim is to rehabilitate the patient back to his near normal or normal lifestyle. ADL assessment is very important tool of assessment to identify the functional disability.

An ADL assessment is simply an assessment to analyze a person's ability to perform his/her personel care and general activities, which he/she need to do on a routine basis in and around home.

Physiotherapist by assessing the ADL assessment, determines the level and type of assistance a person requires in order to live an independent life as possible.

This assessment will also ables the therapist to plan for the modifications that the patient may be deemed necessary for making him independent.

What are the areas to assess for ADL?

BASIC ADL

- Self-care activities
- Mobility
- Communication

Self-Care

- Feeding
- Grooming
- Dressing
- Bathing
- Toilet activities

Mobility

- Bed mobility
- Wheelchair mobility
- Transfers from bed to wheelchair and vice versa
- Ambulation

Communication

- Writing skills
- Speaking
- Using various communication devises like telephone, mobile, etc.

Feeding: Assess the patient how he/she is feeding, the type of set up, utensils and spoons used, ability to chew and swallow.

Grooming and hygiene: Assess how the patient is able to do or how far he need assistance in oral care, hair dressing, bathing, shaving, etc.

Dressing: Assess the patient, her/his ability to wear the clothes, buttoning, lacing the shoes, buckling the belt, etc.

There are many scales available to assess the ADL performance of the patient. To brief FIM (Functional independent measure) can be used.

It has the following rubic measurements:

- 7—independent
- 6—modified independent
- 5—supervision/set up modification
- 4—minimal assistance
- 3—moderate assistance
- 2—maximal assistance
- 1—total assistance

Apart from this, an evidence-based assessment can also be done by Barthel Index, Katz index of independence in ADL, etc.

14 Psychological Assessment

What is Psychological Assessment?

It is also known as mental status examination which is a component of all medical assessments which is psychological equivalent of physical assessment in evaluations.

It is very important in the neurological and psychiatric evaluation of the patients.

Why Psychological Assessment is needed?

It is important to evaluate the mental status of the patient both quantitatively and qualitatively in order to assess how the present pathology has its effect on the psychological status of the patient. It is proven that a sound mind leads to sound body, and almost many neurological disorders have the recovery factor depending on the mental status also.

What should be Known?

To have a proper mental status examination, it is important to have some understanding of the patient's social, cultural and educational background.

What should be Assessed?

The most detailed assessment of the mental status or psychological evaluation should include information about:

- General appearance of the patient
- Level of motor activity
- Speech
- Thought process
- Thought content
- Perception skills
- Intellect skill
- Insight

Appearance: Age, sex, race, body built, posture, eye contact, dress, grooming manner, attentiveness towards examiner, distinguishing features, prominent physical abnormalities, emotional facial expressions should be assessed

Motor: Retardation, agitation, abnormal movements, gait catatonia should be assessed

Speech: Rate, rhythm, volume, amount, articulation, spontaneity.

Affect: Stability, range, appropriateness, intensity, affect, mood.

Thought content: Check for any suicidal ideation, death wishes, homicidal ideation, depressive cognitions, obsessions, ruminations, phobias, ideas of reference, paranoid ideation, magical ideations, delusions, overvalued ideas.

Thought process: Associations, coherence, logic, blocking, attention skills are assessed.

Perception: Check for any hallucinations, illusions depersonalization, deja vu, etc.

Intellect: Assess the global impression— average, above average or below average.

Insight: Awareness of illness and reaction to it.

EVIDENCE-BASED PRACTICE

For evidence-based practice, the following scales can be used for psychological assessment of the patient:

1. Mini-mental scale
2. Cognitive capacity screening examination
3. HADS

Balance and Coordination

BALANCE

When an individual is able to maintain a position for certain interval of time, it is called balance.

Sensory organs, like eyes, ears, play an important role in maintaining a balance.

Various tests are first explained and demonstrated to the patient and then asked to repeat them accordingly.

Mainly Berg balance scale is used to assess the balance of an individual.

a. Sitting to standing.
b. Standing unsupported.
c. Sitting with back unsupported but feet supported on the ground.
d. Standing to sit.
e. Standing unsupported with eyes closed.
f. Standing unsupported with feet together.
g. Turn 360 degrees.

Various tests of balance are as follows:

1. **Romberg test:** Here therapist instructs patient to stand straight with both feet together with eyes open and close. Therapist should stand adjacent to the patient so that the patient should not fall. This test is positive if patient sways side-to-side or front and back with closed eyes.

2. **Single leg standing:** Here therapist instructs the individual to stand on one leg with eyes open and close. On eye closing, if patient sways in this position side-to-side or front and back, then the test is positive.

3. **Alternate single leg standing:** Here therapist instructs the patient to stand on single leg alternatively with eyes open and close. If patient falls down with close eyes, then the test is positive.

4. **Wobble board:** Here therapist instructs the patient to stand on a wobble board and start moving the board on right and left side. If patient is able to maintain himself from falling down, it improves his/her balance.

COORDINATION

When an individual is able to perform rhythmic, controlled, accurate movement against a motor response, then it is known as coordination.

If a person is not able to perform movement in a rhythmic, controlled way, it is called in-coordination.

Conditions that represent incoordination are as follows:

1. Cerebral palsy (CP)
2. Huntington's disease
3. Parkinsonism
4. Traumatic brain injury (TBI)
5. Brain tumors
6. Stroke

Various coordination tests are as follows:

1. **Finger nose test:** Here therapist instructs the patient to bring the finger towards his nose and try to touch it smoothly.

2. **Finger to examiner's finger:** Here therapist instructs the patient to touch therapist finger with his finger tip smoothly.

3. **Alternate finger nose test:** Here therapist instructs the patient to touch the nose with all the fingers that is starting with index finger to little finger.

4. **Heel shin test:** Here therapist instructs the patient to slide the heel of one leg on the shin of other leg. This test is performed suitably in supine position.

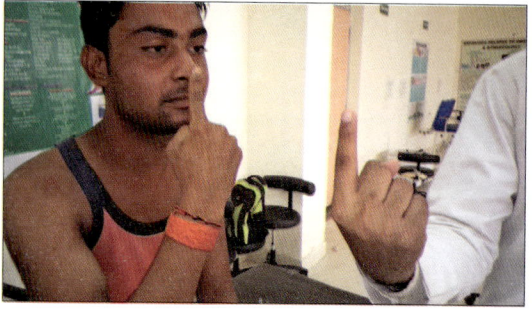 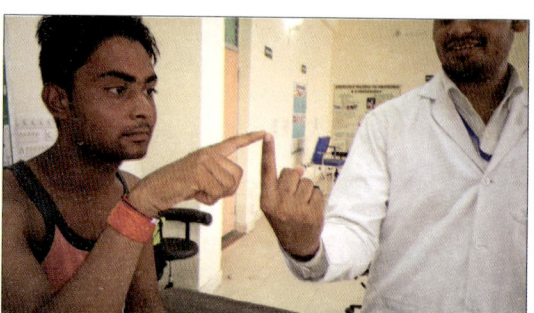

Finger nose test

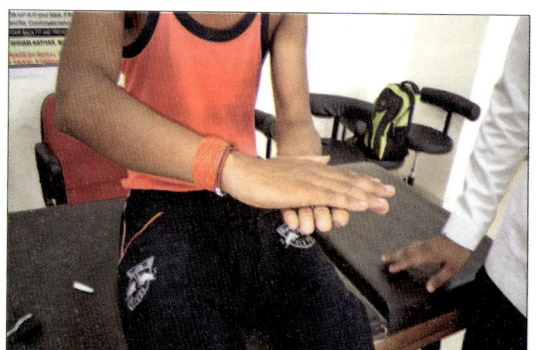 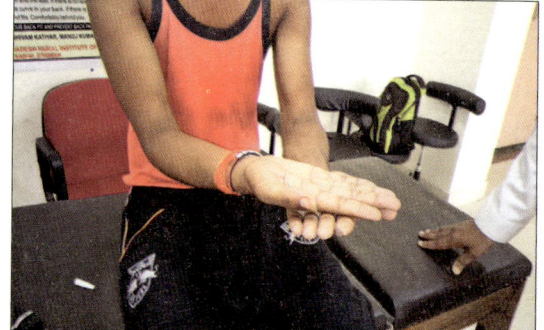

Alternative movements

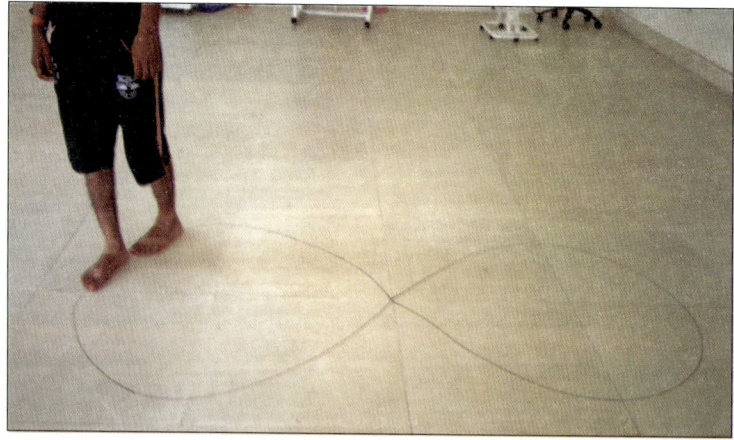

Walking on figure of eight

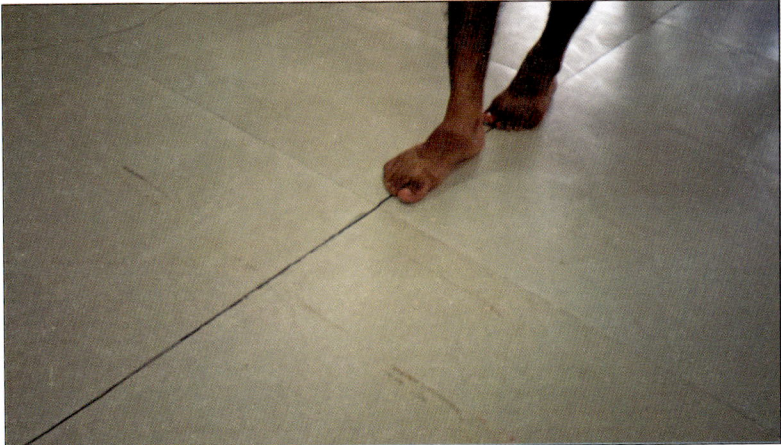

Walking on a straight line

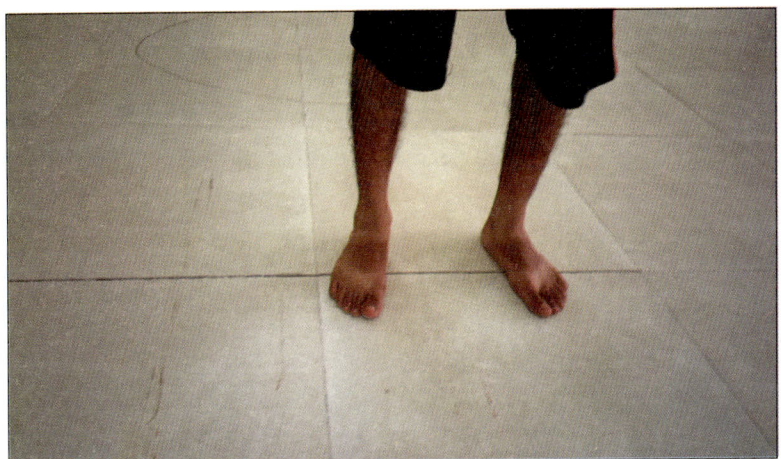

Walking on straight line sideways

5. **Circle drawing test with upper limb:** Here therapist instructs the patient to draw a circle with extended arm in supine, standing and sitting positions. The movement should be smooth in nature.

6. **Circle drawing test with lower limb:** Here therapist instructs the patient to draw a circle with extended leg in supine, and standing positions. The movement should be smooth in nature.

7. **Tandem walk:** Here therapist instructs the patient to put the heel of one foot immediately in front of toes of other foot.

8. **Hurdle clearing test:** Here therapist arranges some sticks, brick pieces or any object in straight line or zig-zag manner. Later he instructs the patient to cross the objects placed on the floor without touching them.

9. **Alternate box walk:** Here boxes of alternate shades are drawn by the therapist on the floor. Patient is instructed to put the leg on the boxes of alternate shades as he walks over them. Patient has to prevent him/her self from falling or keeping the leg outside the shaded box.

10. **Figure of eight walk:** Here two circles adjacent to each other like number eight are marked on the floor. Therapist instructs the patient to walk on the marked figure of eight in a slow rhythmic way.

16

Musculoskeletal System Assessment

SUBJECTIVE

Name:
Dominance:
Address:
Residence: Ground/Upper
Socioeconomic status :
Age: Sex:
Occupation   :
Chief complaints   :
    According to the chronological order
    (Major problems comes first)

………………………………………………
………………………………………………........

HISTORY

Past Medical History

Any previous history of same problem

Present Medical History

Onset   : Sudden/gradual
Duration   :
Side   :
Associated problem   : Problems other than the
                     primary one

Personal History

Family History

OBJECTIVE ASSESSMENT

On Observation

Posture

Levels of ear   : Equal/unequal
Levels of shoulder   : Equal/unequal
Levels of ASIS   : Equal/unequal

Gait   Normal/abnormal

External Appliances

- Splints   • Braces   • Bandages

On Palpation

Muscle tone   : Increased/decreased
Skin temperature
Abnormal prominence

Edema

Location/generalized/localized/pitting/non-pitting/endurated/non-endurated

On Examination

Vital signs

Blood pressure   : 120/80 mm Hg
Temperature   : 98.6°F
Respiratory rate   : 16–18 cycles/minute
Heart rate   : 72–80 beats/minute

Measurements

1. Limb length
2. Limb girth
3. Assessment of tone and power

Movements

Joint range of motion asessment
ADL assessment

Special tests

Investigations
Diagnosis
Problem listing
Physiotherapy management

17

Measurement of Range of Motion (Goniometry)

Measuring the range of motion is a routine and mandatory procedure for musculoskeletal assessment. It is a basic skill to be learned by the physiotherapist for measuring the range of motion of various joints. Even though there are many advanced measurement techniques available today, the *goniometry* is still reliable and a simple way of measuring the joint range of motion.

The technique to measure joint range of motion is called goniometry. The instrument used to measure joint ROM is goniometer.

Goniometry is used in the following:

- To know the joint range of motion.
- To assess joint pathology.
- To measure the prognosis as a part of evidence-based practice.
- Used in biofeedback.

A goniometer consists of:

- A stable or fixed arm.
- A movable arm.
- Fulcrum.
- Protractor.
- Marker or pointer.

There are various types of goniometers available today.

- Long lever goniometer.
- Short lever goniometer.
- Finger goniometer
- Bulb goniometer.
- Electro-goniometer (El-Gon).

Goniometry measurements are done by two ways:

1. Active goniometry: In this, the patient himself moves his joint and the therapist measures the range.

2. Passive goniometry: In some conditions where the patient cannot move his limb by himself, the therapist moves the limb passively and measures the range.

PRINCIPLES OF GONIOMETRY

- It must be practiced in a well-ventilated room.
- Patient must be completely relaxed in a suitable position and should be explained the entire procedure.
- Tight clothing which restrict the movement must be stripped off or loosened.
- Avoid errors in taking readings.
- The fulcrum should not move and must be fixed at same point throughout the range.
- Take care to see that arms of goniometer do not impinge patient's body.
- The entire procedure should not be painful.
- Suitable position is necessary to measure and hence needs patient's cooperation.

TECHNIQUES

1. Place the patient in a suitable position.
2. Place the fulcrum on joint axis.
3. Fix the fulcrum.
4. Place the movable arm on the mobile segment to be measured.
5. Place the stable arm on other side.
6. Now, ask the patient to move in full range, gently move the movable arm along.
7. Mark the markings on the body, if necessary.
8. Take the readings by angle formed over the protractor.

Joint	Movement	Position of patient and fulcrum (axis)	Movable arm	Stable arm	Normal range
Shoulder	Flexion	Attain a supine position for the patient with arm lying side of the patient. *Fulcrum:* Center of the humeral head at the level of acromion process.	Aligned with midline of the humerus parallel to the arm. Use a skin marker and draw a line, if required.	Parallel to mid-axillary line. Draw a line with skin marker, if required	0–167° (American Academy of Orthopedic Surgeons) +/–4.7°
	Extension	Attain a prone position for the patient. Provide a nose gap. Arm resting side of the body *Fulcrum:* Center of the humeral head near acromion process.	Same as above	Same as above	0–62° (American Academy of Orthopedic Surgeons)
	Abduction	Make the patient supine lying with arm resting on the side of the body *Fulcrum:* Over the tip of coracoid process.	Parallel to the humerus	Below the clavicle parallel to it	184°+/–7° (American Academy of Orthopedic Surgeons)
	Internal rotation	Make the patient lie supine at the edge of the couch/bed with shoulder 90° abducted, forearm neutral and elbow flexed at 90°. *Fulcrum:* Over the olecranon process	Aligned with ulna parallel to styloid process.	Aligned vertically	69°+/–4.6° (American Academy of Orthopedic Surgeons)
	External rotation	Same as above	Same as above	Same as above	104°+/–8.5° (American Academy of Orthopedic Surgeons)
Elbow	Flexion	Make the patient lie supine at the edge of the couch/bed. Shoulder neutral with arm at side, forearm supinated. *Fulcrum:* Lateral epicondyle of humerus.	Parallel to radius styloid process	Aligned parallel with humerus	0–141° +/–4.9° (American Academy of Orhtopedic Surgeons)
	Extension	Same as above	Same as above	Same as above	0.3° +/–2° (American Academy of Orthopedic Surgeons)
Wrist	Flexion	Make the subject in sitting position with forearm stabilize on the supporting surface (use a table or pillow) *Fulcrum:* Lateral wrist over the triquetrum.	Aligned parallel to the fifth metacarpal laterally	Aligned parallel to the lateral side of the ulna	75°+/–6.6° (American Academy of Orthopedic Surgeons)
	Extension	Same as above	Same as above	Same as above	74°+/–6.6° (American Academy of Orthopaedic Surgeons)

Contd.

Joint	Movement	Position of patient and fulcrum (axis)	Movable arm	Stable arm	Normal range
	Radial deviation	Make the subject sitting with forearm resting on the table *Fulcrum:* Capitate (dorsally)	Aligned with metacarpal of the middle finger dorsally.	Aligned with dorsal aspect of the forearm	21°+/−4.0° (American Academy of Orthopedic Surgeons)
	Ulnar deviation	Same as above	Same as above	Same as above	35°+/−3.8° (American Academy of Orthopedic Surgeons)
Metacarpophalangeal joint (MCP)	Flexion	Make the subject sitting with forearm supported completely on a table *Fulcrum:* Dorsal metacarpophalangeal joint	Aligned with the proximal phalange	Aligned with the corresponding metacarpal	86° index, 91° ring finger, 105° little finger.
	Extension	Make the subject sitting with forearm completely resting on a table *Fulcrum:* Dorsal MCP joint	Aligned with the proximal phalange	Aligned with the metacarpal	22° index, 18° long, 23° ring, 19° little (American Academy of Orthopedic Surgeons)
	Abduction	Subject sitting with forearm resting on table *Fulcrum:* Dorsal MCP joint	Aligned with proximal phalange	Aligned with metacarpal	
Lower limb					
Hip joint	Flexion	Subject is in supine lying *Fulcrum:* Greater trochanter	Aligned with the femur laterally	Aligned with the trunk laterally	
	Extension	Same as above	Same as above	Same a above	
	Medial rotation	Subject is in sitting position with hip knee flexion on a table *Fulcrum:* Tibial tuberosity	Shin of tibia	Vertical to the movable arm	
	Lateral rotation	Same as above	Same as above	Same as above	
	Abduction	Patient is supine lying with lower limbs parallel to each other *Fulcrum:* ASIS	Movable arm is parallel to the femur shaft anteriorly	Stable arm on the imaginary line joining the two ASIS	
	Adduction	Same as above	Same as above	Same as above	
Knee joint	Flexion	Patient sitting on a high stool, foot off the ground *Fulcrum:* Lateral tibial condyle	Movable arm parallel to the fibula laterally	Stable arm parallel to the femur	
	Extension	Same as above	Same as above	Same as above	
Ankle	Dorsiflexion	Patient sitting on a high stool, foot off the ground *Fulcrum:* Lateral malleolus	Movable arm para-llel to the lateral surface of the foot	Stable arm parallel to the leg	
	Plantar flexion	Same as above	Same as above	Same as above	
Subtalar joint	Inversion and eversion	Please see below for complete description			

MEASUREMENT OF INVERSION AND EVERSION

1. Mark a point with a chalk or marker on the floor.
2. Make the patient step on it such that his heel is exactly on the point.
3. Now mark a point on the floor exactly in front of the second toe of the foot.
4. Now ask the patient to do inversion.
5. Now again mark in front of the second toe in inverted position.
6. Ask the patient to come to neutral position.
7. Now ask the patient to do eversion.
8. Again mark a point on floor infront of the second toe.
9. Now join the points, angle is formed, measure it with goniometer.
10. Kindly see below for a pictorial demonstration.

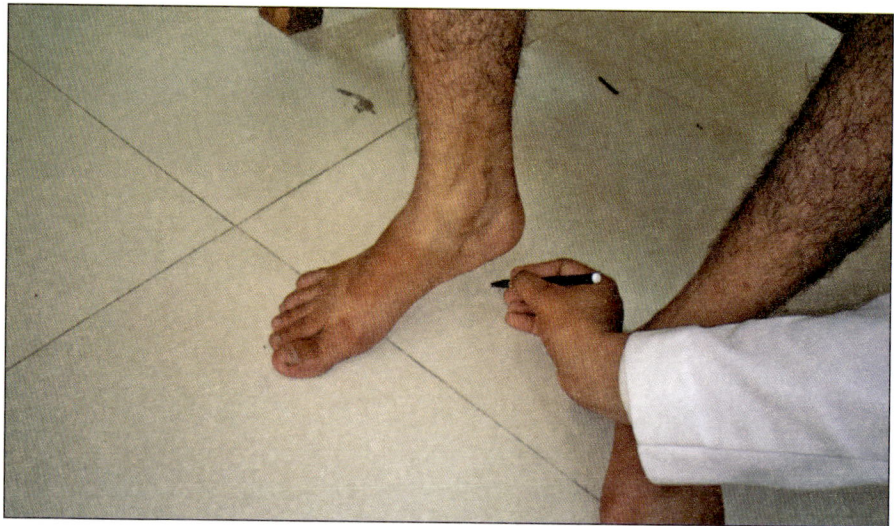

Step 1: Mark a point under the heel of the patient.

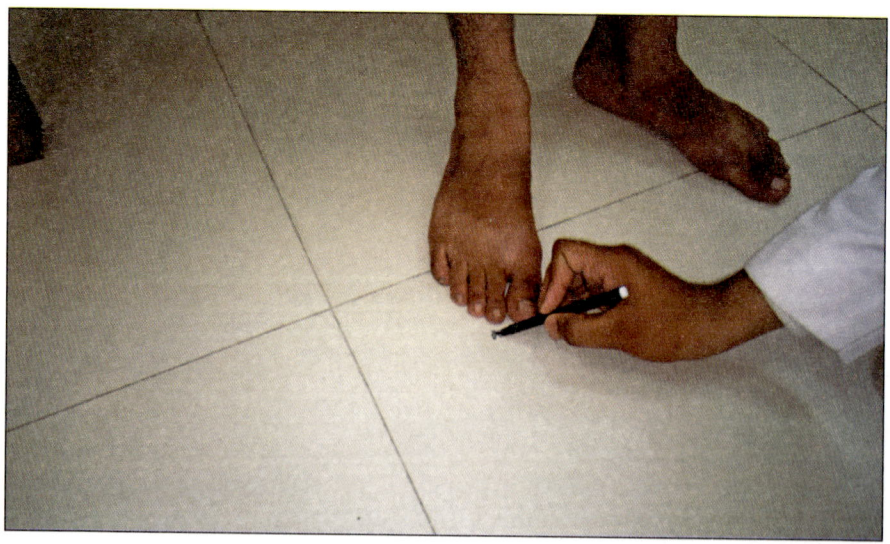

Step 2: Mark a point infront of the second toe.

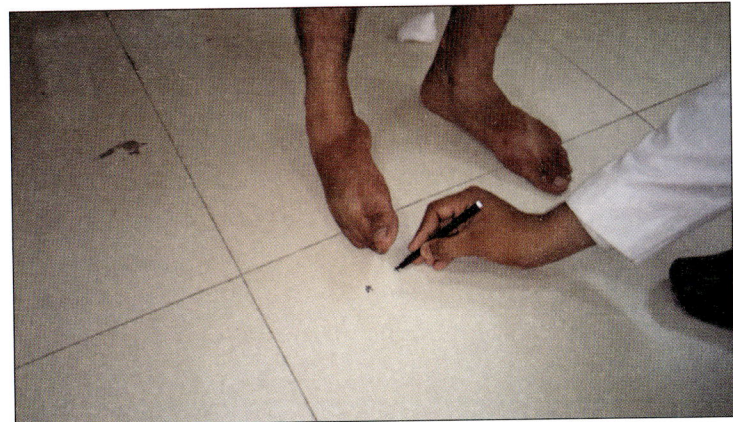

Step 3: Ask the patient to perform inversion

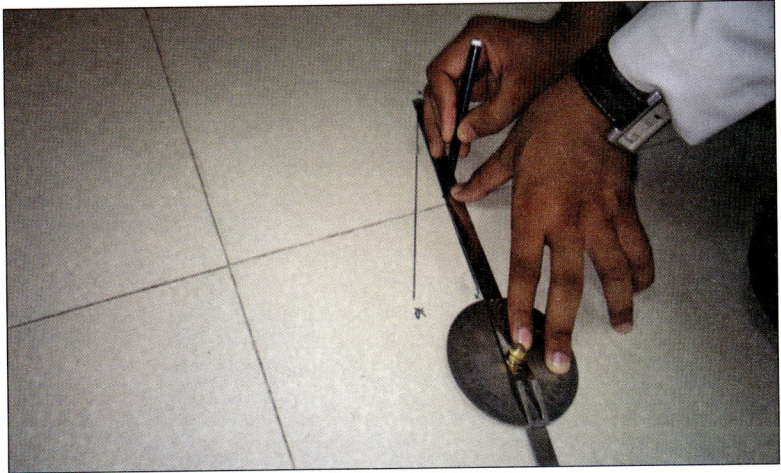

Step 4: Now joint the points to make an angle

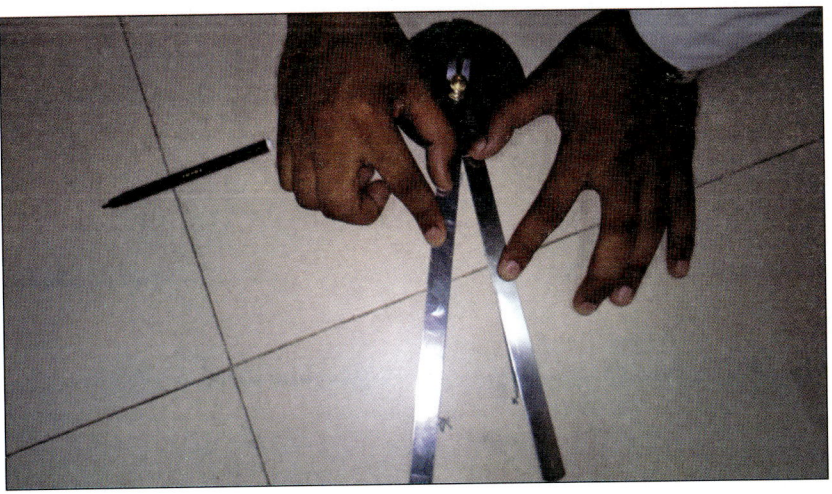

Step 5: Now with the help of goniometer, measure the angle formed

Joint	Movement	Position of patient and fulcrum (axis)	Movable arm	Stable arm	Normal range
Cervical spine					
Cervical	Flexion	Patient is in sitting position with thoracic and lumbar spine supported *Fulcrum:* External auditory meatus.	Aligned with the tip of the nose	Aligned vertically with movable arm.	65–70° (American Academy of Orthopedic Surgeons)
	Extension	Same as above	Same as above	Same as above	64.5–70° (American Academy of Orthopedic Surgeons)
	Lateral rotation	Patient is in sitting position with thoracic and lumbar spine supported *Fulcrum:* Center of the head	Aligned with the tip of the nose	Aligned with the acromion process	77.5+/-7.50 (American Academy of Orthopedic Surgeons)
	Lateral flexion	Patient is in sitting posing with thoracic and lumbar spine supported *Fulcrum:* C7 spinous process	Aligned with midline passing through the external occipital protuberance	Aligned parallel with the thoracic spine	40–48° (American Academy of Orthopedic Surgeons)
Thoraco-lumbar	Lateral flexion	Patient is in standing position. *Fulcrum:* S1 spinous process	Aligned with the C7 spinous process.	Aligned vertically with the movable arm.	25° (American Academy of Orthopedic Surgeons)
	Rotation	Patient is in sitting position. *Fulcrum:* Center of the head.	Aligned with the ASIS.	Aligned with acromion process.	45° (American Medical Association)

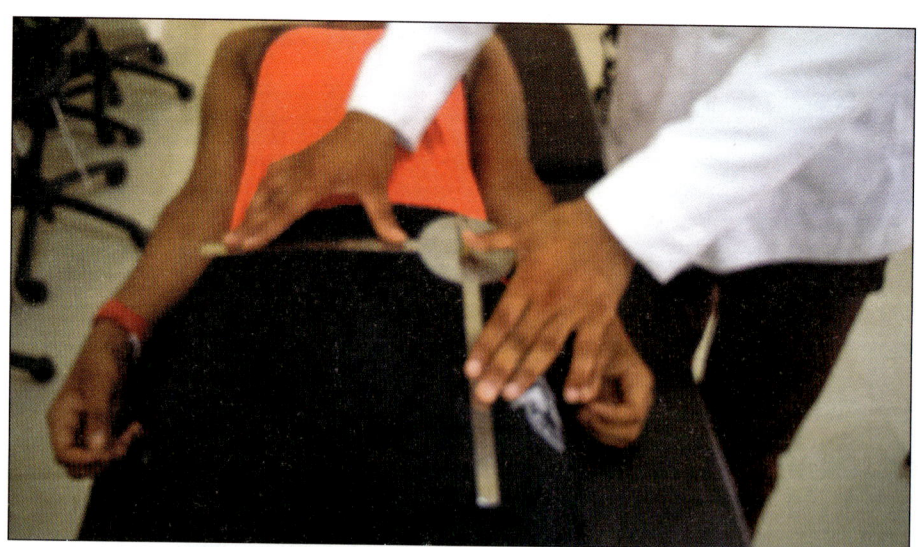

Hip abduction

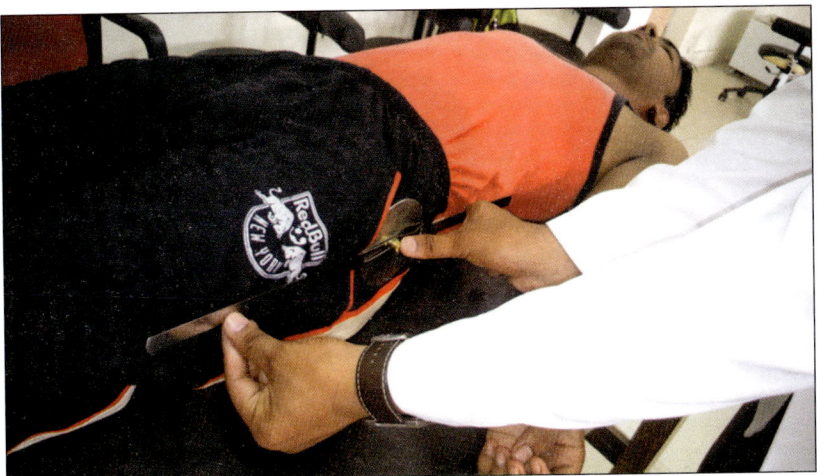

Hip flexion

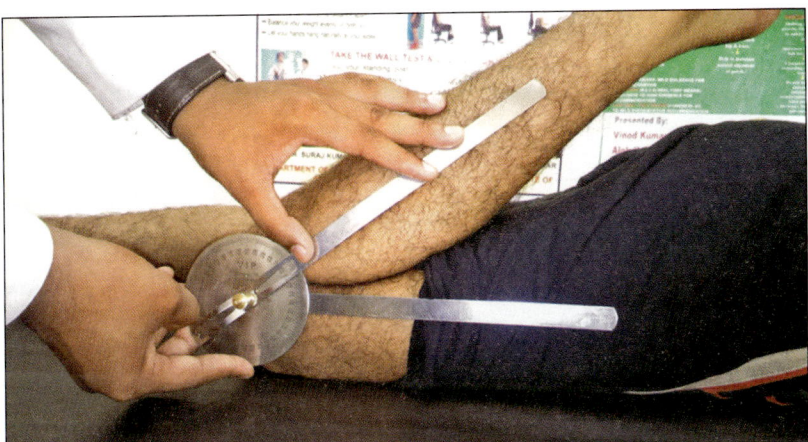

Knee flexion

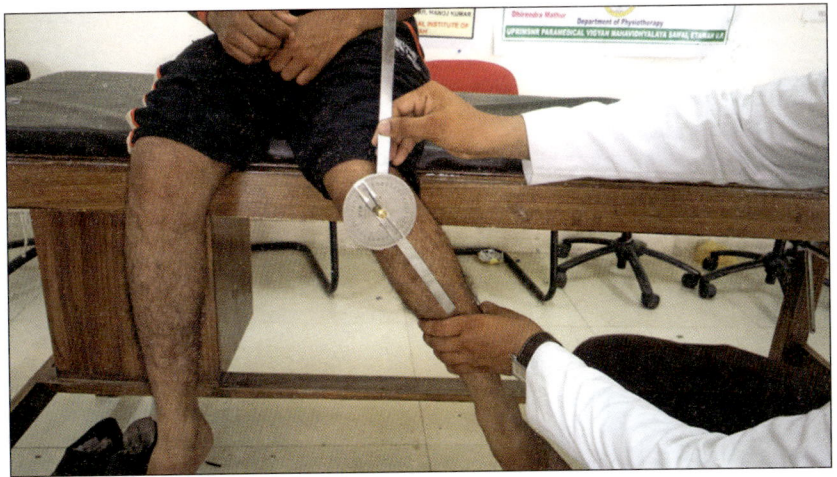

Hip medial rotation

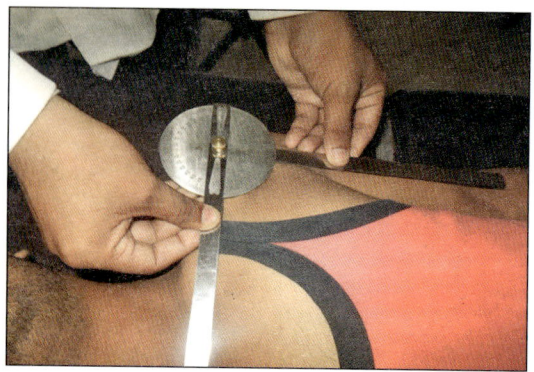

Shoulder abduction

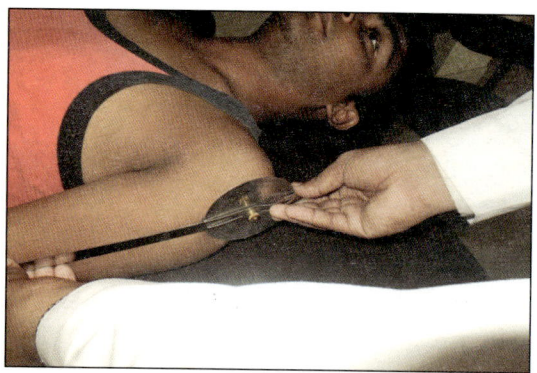

Shoulder flexion

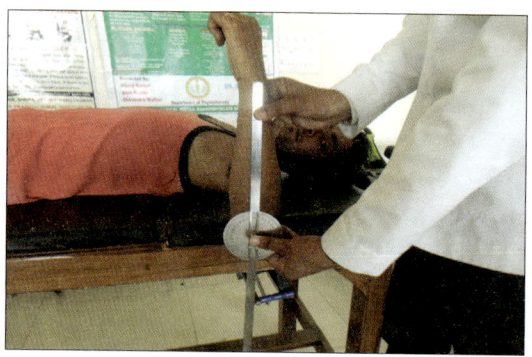

Shoulder medial and lateral rotation

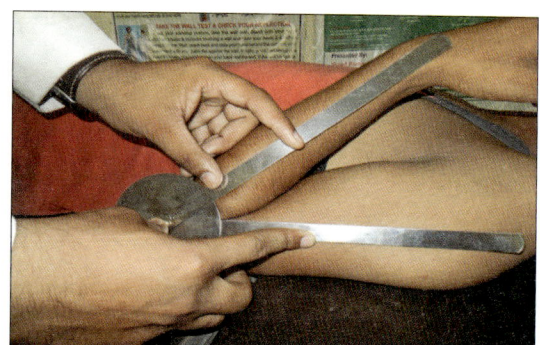

Elbow flexion

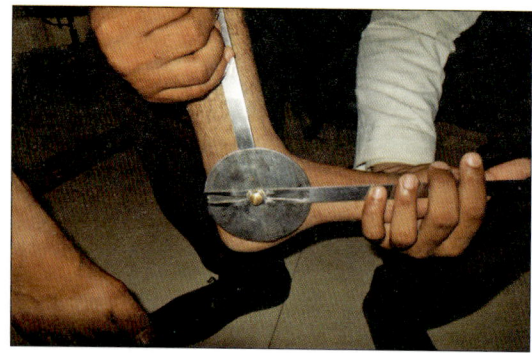

Ankle dorsiflexion

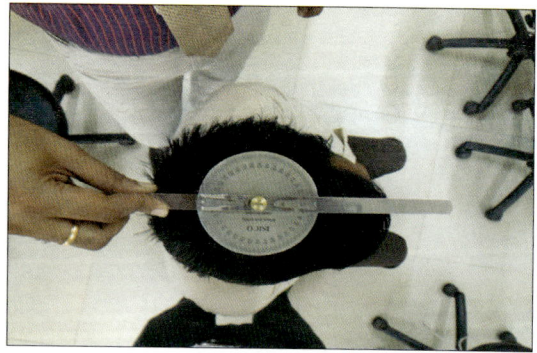

Cervical rotation

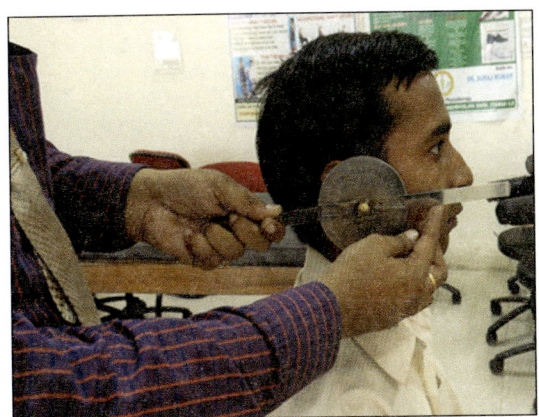
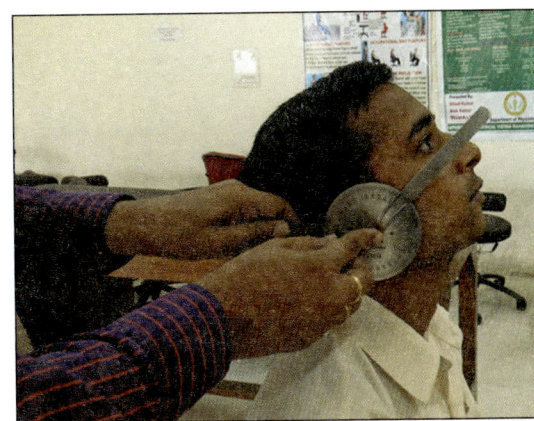

Cervical extension

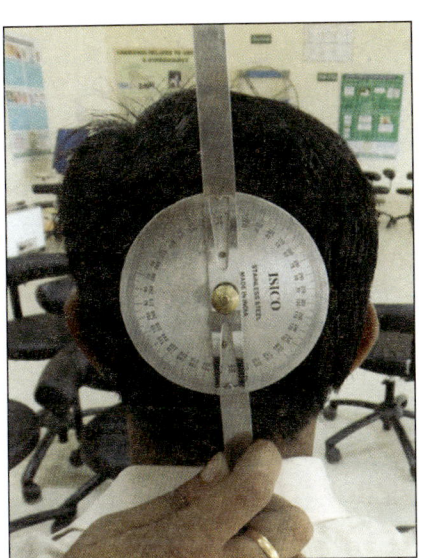
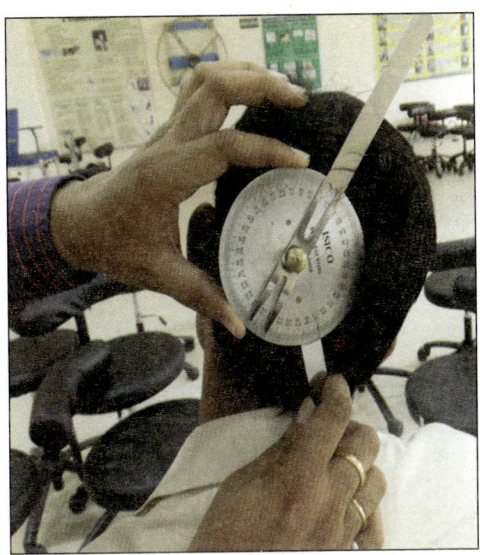

Cervical lateral flexion

18

Limb Length Measurements

Measurements of the length of whole or a segment of the limb are done to detect shortening or lengthening of the limb.

It is an important part of clinical examination.

Anatomical markings to be noted for measurement:

1. Umbilicus
2. Anterior superior iliac spine (ASIS)
3. Greater trochanter
4. Tibial tuberosity
5. Lateral epicondyle
6. Medial malleolus
7. Lateral malleolus

TYPES OF MEASUREMENT

1. Apparent length
2. True length

Apparent Length

1. The measurement is made with the limbs in deformed position of abduction or adduction.
2. Apparent shortening is the result of muscular weakness or spasticity; inother words due to muscular imbalances.

Technique

1. Make the patient lie down in supine.
2. Ask the patient to relax.

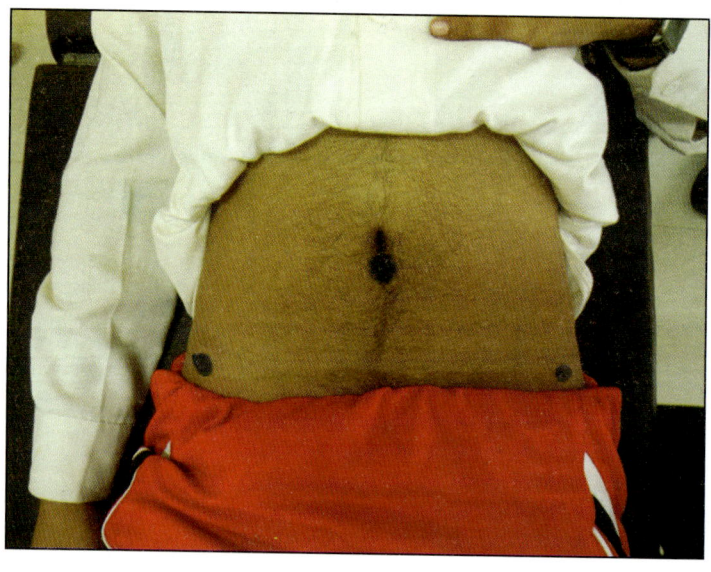

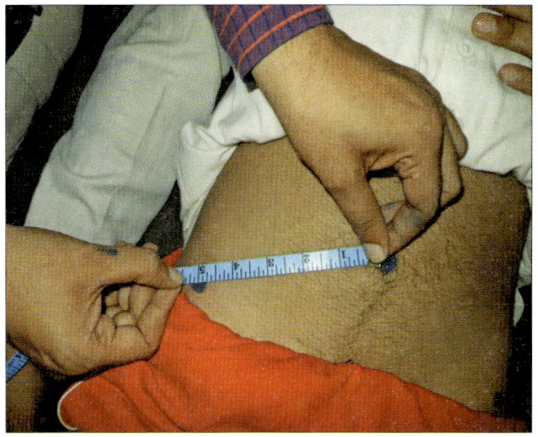
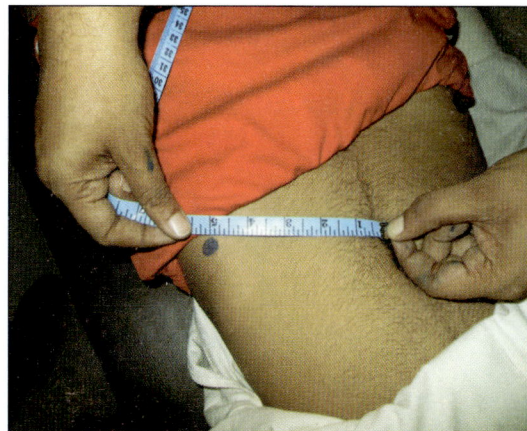

3. Explain the procedure to the patient, take consent.

4. Expose the part to be measured by having privacy.

5. Note the markings at umbilicus and medial malleolus.

6. Now with the help of inch tape, measure the length from umbilicus to medial malleolus of the affected leg.

7. Measure the length from umbilicus to medial malleolus of normal limb.

8. Compare the measurements.

True Length

1. Meausurement is taken after squaring of pelvis.

2. Squaring of the pelvis is done by first measuring the distance from umbilicus to ASIS of normal and then affected leg.

3. Now, adduct or abduct the variable hip joint to the point where the distance between umbilicus and ASIS of both sides is equal.

4. Now the measurement is taken from ASIS to medial malleolus of normal and affected limb.

5. Compare the measurements.

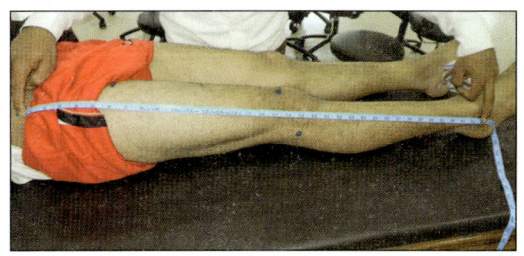

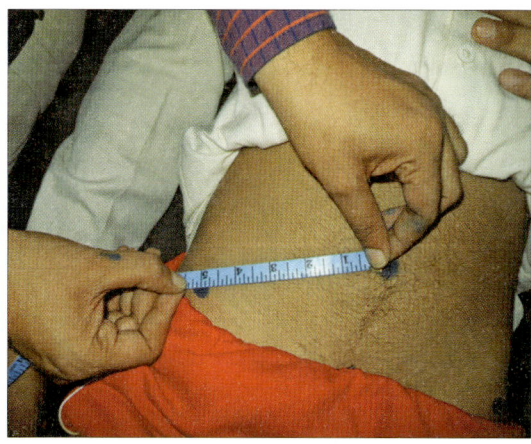

19

Limb Girth Measurements

LIMB GIRTH

It is the circumference or thickness or diameter of the limb.

Girth or circumference of the limb gets affected by many factors:

1. Prolonged bed rest
2. Severe tissue or bony damage
3. Deformity
4. Neurological issue

Girth of a limb needs to be assessed to:

1. Compare it with the sound limb
2. Regain the girth similar to the sound limb
3. Regain the strength, endurance similar to that of sound

Apparatus Required

1. Inch tape
2. Non-toxic marker

Methods

Inch Tape Method

Apparatus required:

1. Inch tape
2. Non-toxic marker

Procedure

First the length of *unaffected* limb is measured with the help of inch/measuring tape. The total length is divided in 3 parts with help of a non-toxic marker. Readings are recorded.

Then the *affected* limb is measured with the help of inch/measuring tape. The total length is divided in 3 parts with help of a non-toxic marker. Readings are recorded.

Volumetric Analysis

Apparatus required:

1. Large glass/metal tub
2. Water

Procedure

Water poured in the large glass or metal tub. Length of the unaffected limb is measured and divided into 3 equal parts with the help of a non-toxic marker. Now the marked part is immersed in water-filled tub and amount of water spilled out of the tub is noted.

Now the affected limb is measured and divided into 3 equal parts with the help of a non-toxic marker. The marked part is immersed in water-filled tub and amount of water spilled out of the tub is noted.

Disadvantage

- Method is strenuous.
- Requires more candidates to perform the activity.
- Patient doesn't cooperate.

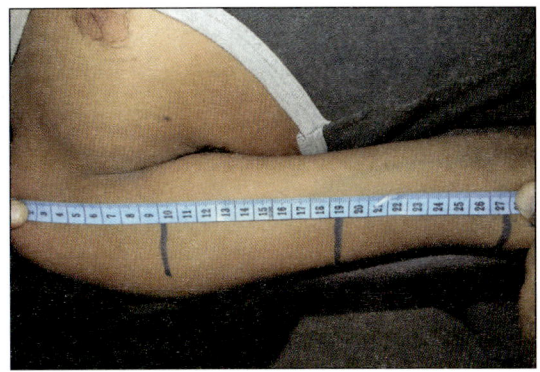
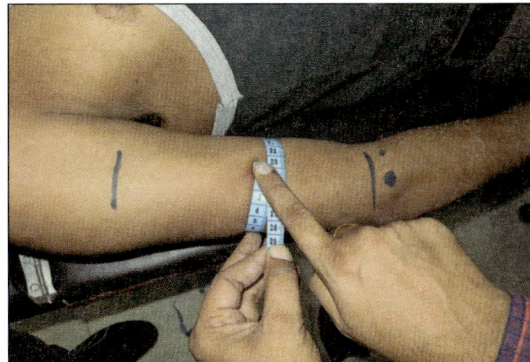

LIMB GIRTH MEASUREMENT OF UPPER LIMB

Arm

- Fixed point: Acromion process
- End point: Lateral epicondyle

Method: Patient is positioned supine in anatomical position. First the unaffected limb is measured and later the affected limb.

Acromion process and lateral epicondyle are marked with non-toxic marker. These points are measured with the help of inch/measuring tape. Measured length is divided in 3 equal parts. Circumference/girth of marked mid-part is measured and readings are recorded.

Forearm

Fixed point: Lateral side of the crease present in the elbow joint on the anterior aspect.
End point: Lower end of radius bone.

Method: Patient is positioned supine in anatomical position. First the unaffected limb is measured and later the affected limb. Lateral side of the crease present in the elbow joint on the anterior aspect is marked with non-toxic marker. Mid of the girth/circumference is measured with an inch tape and the same is recorded.

LOWER LIMB

Thigh

Fixed point: ASIS
End point: Lower end of lateral condyle of femur.

Method: Patient is positioned supine in anatomical position. First the unaffected limb is measured and later the affected limb. Fixed point and end point are marked with non-toxic marker and the mid of thigh is measured with inch tape and readings are recorded.

Leg

Fixed point: Lateral end of fibular head.
End point: Lateral malleoli.

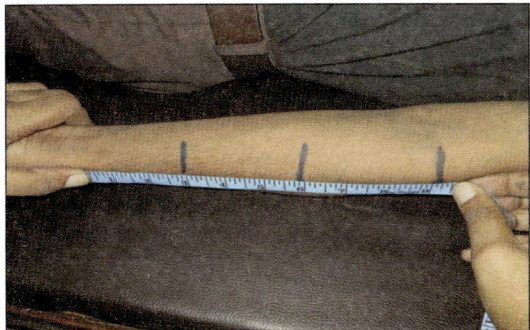
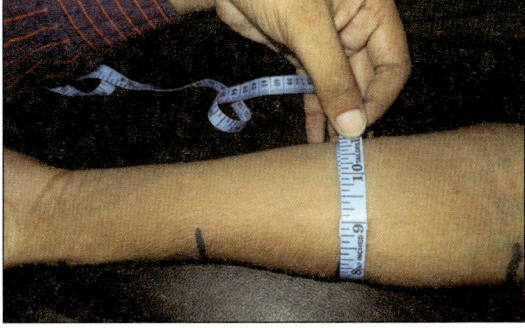

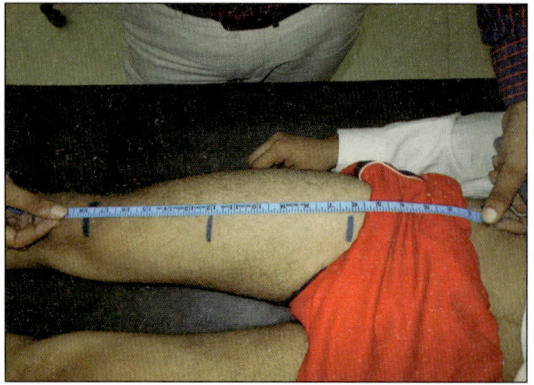 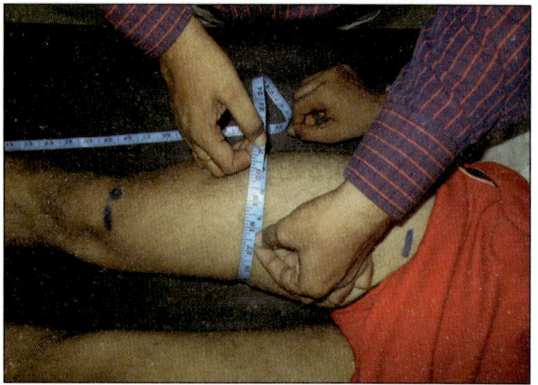

Method: Patient is positioned supine in anatomical position. First the unaffected limb is measured and later the affected limb. Fixed point and end point are marked with non-toxic marker and the mid of leg is measured with inch tape and readings are recorded.

Common Special Tests in Musculoskeletal Assessment

Special Test

These tests are performed by the physiotherapist for the confirmation of the diagnosis.

Lumbar Spine

Test name	Position of the patient	Position of the therapist	Technique	Observation	Remark
1. Slump test	Sitting at the edge of table	Standing at the side of the table	Patient is asked to bend forward without neck flexion. Later on asked to extend the knee with dorsiflexion while therapist applies pressure over the neck and shoulders.	Pain	Stretch in meninges of the spinal cord
2. Straight leg raise (SLR) test or Lasegue's test	Supine with medial rotation and adduction of hip along with extended knee	Standing at the side of the table	Patient is asked to raise the leg with extended knee. Then instructed to lower the leg in knee extension thereby relieving the pain. Dorsiflexion of ankle provokes the pain.	Excruciating pain at 70°	Disc herniation resulting in lower back pain

Contd.

Test name	Position of the patient	Position of the therapist	Technique	Observation	Remark
3. Brudzinski's sign	Supine with medial rotation and adduction of hip along with extended knee	Standing at the side of the table	Same as SLR test but neck is flexed passively	1. Pain 2. If pain doesn't elicited	dura matter stretch or lesion in spinal cord Hamstring tightness
4. Modified SLR test	Side lying with test leg positioned superiorly along with hip and knee flexed to 90°	Therapist stands at the side of the table	By supporting the pelvis, therapist slowly extends the knee	Pain in lower back	Disc herniation resulting in lower back pain
5. Lhermitt's test or Cross-over sign	Patient in supine lying position	Therapist stands by the side of the table	Leg of the unaffected side is lifted gradually and pain is elicited in opposite leg	Pain	Disc herniation resulting in pain
6. Prone knee bending test	Prone lying	Therapist stands by the side of the table	Flex the knee to the maximum ensuring no hip rotation.	Pain in lumbar region, buttock or posterior thigh	L2, L3 nerve root lesion

Contd.

Test name	Position of the patient	Position of the therapist	Technique	Observation	Remark
7. Bowstring test	Supine lying	Stands towards foot end of the table	Therapist places subject's affected leg on his shoulder girdle with extended knee.	Pain radiating in lumbar area	Sciatic nerve compression
8. One leg standing lumbar extention test (stork standing)	Stands on one leg	Stands behind the patient	Subject extends his/her back while standing on one leg	Pain in back	Stress fracture of pars interarticularis (spondylolisthesis) Scottish dog appearance
9. Stoop's test	Standing or walking		Patient performs brisk walk for hardly 50 m.	Pain in gluteal region and lower limbs	Intermittent claudication
Pelvis					
1. Gapping test	Supine lying	Stands by the side of the couch	Therapist applies pressure over ASIS with arms crossed in downward and outward direction.	Pain in one side buttocks or in posterior aspect of leg	Sprain in SI ligament
2. Approximation test	Side lying	Standing behind the couch	Therapist applies pressure over the upper part of the iliac crest in a downward direction.	Pain in the SI joint	SI joint lesion.
3. Sacral apex pressure (prone springing) test	Prone lying	Stands by the side of the couch	Therapist applies pressure over the apex of sacrum with the hands.	Pain in the SI joint	SI joint lesion.

Contd.

Test name	Position of the patient	Position of the therapist	Technique	Observation	Remark
4. Gillet's (sacral fixation) test	Standing	Sitting behind the patient	Therapist commands the patient to stand on one leg with other knee flexes to his chest, while places his/her one thumb over PSIS and other over the sacrum.	Placed thumb over the sacrum moves up	SI joint dysfunction.

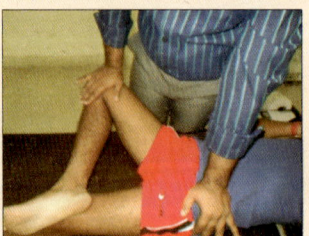

| 5. Genslen's Test | Side lying with upper leg hyper-extended | Standing behind the couch | Therapist asks the patient to hold the lower leg towards the chest. Later while stabilizing the pelvis, therapist extends the hip of the upper leg. | Pain in the sacral region | SI joint lesion |

Hip Joint

| 1. Patrick's or Faber's or figure-of four or Jansen's test | Supine lying | Stands by the side of the couch | Therapist places the test leg over the other extended knee joint by maintaining the position of hip joint in flexion, abduction and external rotation. Slowly therapist applies pressure and tries to lower the knee of test leg towards the edge of the couch. | Knee joint of test leg remains over the extended leg | Spasm of the iliopsoas muscle |

Contd.

Test name	Position of the patient	Position of the therapist	Technique	Observation	Remark
2. Trendelen-burg's test	Standing	Stands behind the patient	Patient is instructed to stand on one leg	Pelvis of the non-stance side drops down	Gluteus medius weakness or unstable hip
3. Thomas test	Supine lying	Stands by the side of the couch	Therapist asks the patient to bring one of the flexed knee toward the chest and looks for the lumbar curve	Extended knee rises off the couch.	Hip flexion contracture
4. J sign	Supine lying	Stands by the side of the couch	Therapist asks the patient to bring one of the flexed knee toward the chest looks for the lumbar curve.	Extended knee abducts	Iliotibial band tightness
5. Kendall test	Supine	Stands by the side of the couch	Therapist instructs the patient to lie supine with knees bent at edge of the couch at 90° and then bring one of the bent knee towards the chest.	Knee hanging at the edge does not remain to 90°	Rectus femoris tightness
6. Ely's test	Prone lying	Stands by the side of the couch	Therapist flexes the knee	On knee flexion, there is flexion of the hip	Rectus femoris tightness

Contd.

Test name	Position of the patient	Position of the therapist	Technique	Observation	Remark
Knee Joint					
1. Abduction or valgus stress test	Supine lying	Stands by the side of the couch	Therapist instructs the patient to be in supine position with knee extended. Then therapist pushes the knee joint from lateral side while maintaining the ankle joint in lateral rotation position with his hands.	Gap will be felt over medial aspect of knee joint	Medial collateral ligament damage (medial instability)
2. Adduction or varus stress test	Supine lying	Stands by the side of the couch	Therapist instructs the patient to be in supine position with knee extended. Then therapist pushes the knee joint from medial side while maintaining the ankle joint in lateral rotation position with his hand.	Gap will be felt over Lateral aspect of knee joint	Lateral collateral ligament damage (lateral instability)
3. Lachman test	Supine lying	Stands by the side of the couch	Therapist holds the knee to be tested in 30° of flexion with one hand while stabilizing the femur with the other. Therapist pushes the condylar part of tibia anteriorly.	Tibia moves anteriorly	Anterior cruciate ligament damage (anterior instability)
4. Drawer sign A	Supine with hip flexion of 45° and knee flexion of 90°	Stands at the foot end of the couch	Therapist holds the foot of the patient in neutral position by sitting over it. He then places his hands around the upper end of tibia and pulls it toward his chest	Tibia moves 6 mm anteriorly	Anterior cruciate ligament damage (anterior instability)

Contd.

Test name	Position of the patient	Position of the therapist	Technique	Observation	Remark
5. Drawer sign B	Supine with hip flexion of 45° and knee flexion of 90°	Stands at the foot end of the couch	Therapist holds the foot of the patient in neutral position by sitting over it. He then places his hands over the upper end of tibia and pushes it posteriorly.	Tibia moves approx. 6 mm posteriorly	Posterior cruciate ligament damage (posterior instability)
6. McMurray test-A	Supine with knee flexed and heel touches the buttocks.	Stands by the side of the couch	Therapist performs medial rotation of tibia with extension of the knee joint.	Pain and click noise in the joint	Lateral meniscus injury or tear
7. McMurray test-B	Supine with knee flexed and heel touches the buttocks	Stands by the side of the couch	Therapist performs lateral rotation of tibia with extension of the knee joint.	Pain and click noise in the joint	Medial meniscus injury or tear
8. Apley's test	Prone lying with knee flexed	Stands by the side of the couch	Therapist fixes the thigh with his knee joint. Then with Distraction, tibia is rotated laterally or medially.	Pain aggrevates	Ligamentous lesion

Contd.

Test name	Position of the patient	Position of the therapist	Technique	Observation	Remark
9. Apley's test	Prone lying with knee flexed	Stands by the side of the couch	Therapist fixes the thigh with his knee joint. Then with compression, tibia is rotated laterally or medially.	Pain aggre-vates	Meniscal injury

Ankle Joint

1. Anterior drawer test of ankle	Supine	Standing at the foot end	Therapist stabilizes both the malleoli with one hand and with other stabilizes the talus. In this position therapist pulls the foot against the gravity while maintaining 20° of plantar flexion.	Pain at the ankle joint	Injury of the anterior talofibular ligament
2. Prone anterior drawer test	Prone lying	Stands at the foot end of the couch	Therapist stabilizes both the malleoli with one hand and with other hand holds the talus and pushes it downwards.	Pain in the ankle joint	Injury of the anterior talofibular ligament

Cervical Spine

1. Foraminal compression test or Spurling's test	Sitting	Stands behind the patient	Patient places the neck in neutral, extension and extension with side flexion position. Therapist applies pressure in above mentioned neck positions.	Pain radiates to the arm to which the head is flexed	Cervical radiculitis

Contd.

Test name	Position of the patient	Position of the therapist	Technique	Observation	Remark
2. Distraction test	Sitting	Stands behind the patient	Therapist places one hand under the chin and other over the occiput and applies traction.	Relieves radiating pain	Relieves radiculating pain
Shoulder Joint					
1. Apprehension (Crank) test	Supine lying	Stands by the head end of the couch	Therapist abducts the arm to 90° and rotates the shoulder laterally. Then he applies downward pressure over the elbow region	Pain in anterior aspect of the glenohumeral joint	Anterior shoulder instability
2. Prone anterior instability test	Prone lying	Stands by the head end of the couch	Therapist abducts the shoulder to 90° and rotates the shoulder laterally. Then he applies downward pressure over humeral head	Pain in the anterior aspect of the GH joint	Anterior shoulder instability
3. Posterior apprehension or stress test	Supine or sitting	Stands by the head end of the couch	Therapist raises the shoulder in plane of the scapula and applies pressure over the elbow joint. At the same time, therapist also horizontally adducts and rotates the arm medially.	Pain in the posterior aspect of the GH joint	Posterior shoulder instability
4. Push or pull test	Supine	Stands by the head end of the couch	Therapist abducts the shoulder to 90° and elbow to 90°. He holds the wrist with one hand and places the other hand over the humeral head. He then pushes the humeral head downward and pulls the wrist upward.	Pain	Posterior shoulder instability

Contd.

Test name	Position of the patient	Position of the therapist	Technique	Observation	Remark
5. Neer impinge- ment test	Sitting	Stands by the side of the patient	Therapist raises and medially rotates the arm.	Pain	Supraspi- natus impingement
6. Speed test	Sittig	Stands by the side of the patient	Patient is instructed to flex the shoulder joint while extending the elbow. Then therapist applies pressure over the wrist in supination and pronation	Pain in the shoulder joint	Bicipital tendinitis
7. Yergason's test	Sitting	Stands by the side of the patient	Therapist instructs the patient to adduct the shoulder and flex elbow to 90° with pronation. Therapist applies pressure while patient is instructed to supinate.	Pain in the anterior aspect of GH joint	Bicipital tendinitis

Contd.

Test name	Position of the patient	Position of the therapist	Technique	Observation	Remark
8. Empty can test	Sitting or standing	Stands by the side of the patient	Patient is instructed to abduct the arm with medial rotation. Therapist applies pressure against the abduction.	Pain in the shoulder joint	Tear in the supraspinatus muscle
9. Roos test	Standing	Infront of the patient	Patient is instructed to abduct both shoulder to 90° with elbow flexed to 90° and then asked to make fist and open it for 3 min.	Unable to maintain the shoulder and elbow position	Thoracic outlet syndrome
Elbow Joint					
1. Lateral epicodylitis (tennis elbow)	Sitting	Stands in front of the patient	Therapist places his thumb over patient's lateral epicondyle and instructs him to make fist with forearm pronated. Then pressure is applied over the wrist during its extension and radial deviation.	Pain over lateral epicondyle	Tennis elbow

Contd.

Test name	Position of the patient	Position of the therapist	Technique	Observation	Remark
2. Golfer's elbow or medial epicodylitis	Sitting	Stands in front of the patient	Therapist places his thumb over patient's medial epicondyle and instructs him to extend elbow and wrist while pressing the medial epicondyle.	Pain over medial epicondyle	Golfer's elbow
3. Tinnel's sign	Sitting	Stands in front of the patient	Therapist tap over the groove (medial epicondyle and olecranon process) on ulnar nerve	Tingling sensation over the course of the nerve from elbow to distal end of hand	Ulnar nerve compression

Wrist Joint

Test name	Position of the patient	Position of the therapist	Technique	Observation	Remark
1. Finkelstein test	Sitting	Stands in front of the patient	Patient is instructed to make fist with thumb inside the fingers. Therapist deviates the fist toward ulnar side.	Pain over tendons extensor pollicis brevis and abductor pollicis longus.	De-Quervain's disease
2. Phalen's test	Sitting	Stands in front of the patient	Therapist instructs the patient to flex both the wrist joints with fingers extended.	Tingling sensation in thumb, index, middle and lateral half of the ring finger	Median nerve compression

21

Obstetrics and Gynecology Assessment

The assessment includes two divisions:
1. Subjective assessment
2. Objective assessment

SUBJECTIVE ASSESSMENT

It includes, introduction of the patient, chief complaints and history taking.

Introduction of the patient: Take the name of the patient. Age, occupation, address, socio-economic status of the patient.

LMP (*last menstrual period*): Record the date of LMP.

If in case of primigravida, also record EDD (estimated date of delivery).

Menstrual history: Take a detailed menstrual history including the type of flow, regularity, pain and clots.

Marital history: Take the marital history of the patient. Ask the date of marriage, and whether the marriage is consanguineous.

Obstetric History

Take a detailed history of trimesters including the symptoms of pregnancy.

General Health

- BMI assessment and assess for obesity
- Hormonal status and influence
- Any complaints of pain
- Current medications and their effects
- History or complaint of incontinence

Medical history: Check for diabetis, hypertension or any other medical complications.

OBJECTIVE ASSESSMENT

Assessing pelvic floor muscles strength:
- Make the patient lie supine. Take consent of the patient. Explain the entire procedure. Have privacy.
- Assess the pelvic floor muscle strentgth by vaginal weights such as femina cones.

Assessing for Diastasis Recti

- Make the patient lie in a crook lying position.
- Ask the patient to relax completely and have a normal breath.
- Explain the entire procedure to the patient.
- Take the consent from the patient and have privacy.
- Now ask the patient to raise her shudders and head off the floor and reach the hands to knee.
- The therapist shall keep the hand on the midline over the linea alba to palpate the abdominal contractions.
- When the patient actively contracts the abdominal muscle, if the therapist feels the gap in the midline, then the test is positive.

POSTURE ANALYSIS

Make the patient stand. Observe the patient posture from lateral, anterior and posterior views. Analyze the posture and report in the following table below. Report any postural deviations observed. Check whether the postural deviations are fixed or malleable. Also find out the reason for the changes, e.g. due to pregnancy (physiological) or neurological, musculoskeletal defect (pathological).

Area to be observed	Lateral view	Anterior view	Posterior view
Head			
Shoulders			
Mid/upper back			
Abdomen			
Low back			
Knees			
Ankles			

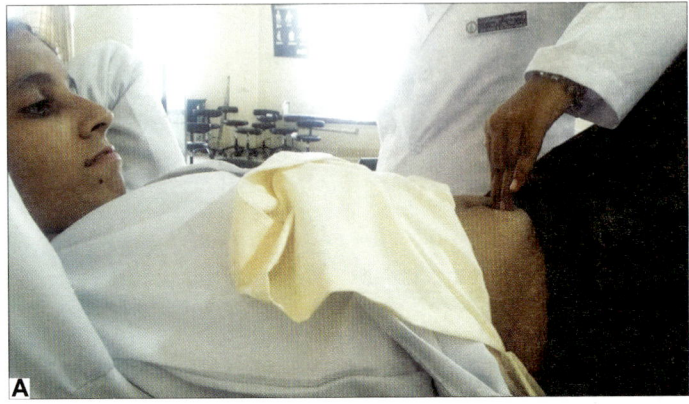

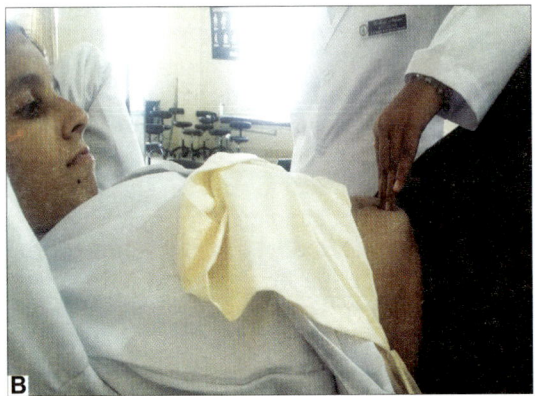

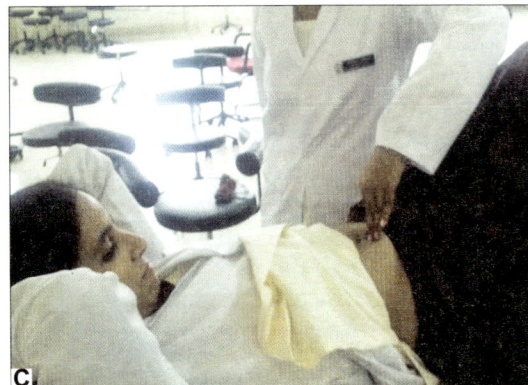

Checking for diastasis recti

RANGE OF MOTION

- Assess the mobility of all joints (Refer goniometry section).
- Apart from the above assessment, also analyze the muscle strength of all myotomes.
- Assess for reflexes and find out the abnormal reflexes

GAIT ANALYSIS

- Check the step length, stride length, cadence.
- Check whether there is arm swing or not.
- Check whether the pattern of gait is normal or any deviations present.

INVESTIGATIONS

- Investigations depends upon the chief complaints of the patient.
- In case of diastasis recti, an EMG may be required.
- In case of incontinence, urine examination, culture and sensitivity may be required.

22

Pediatric Assessment

Evaluation Form

Name : _____

Age: _____ Sex: _____

Socioeconomic status: _____

Address: _____

_____

_____

Dominence: _____

HISTORY
(TAKEN FROM MOTHER/CARETAKER)

Prenatal:

Perinatal:

Postnatal:

On observation:

Dysmorphic features:

Supine Observation

- Attitutde at rest
- Symmetry of the body
- Involuntary movements
- Position of the head
- Visual fixation and tracking
- Attitutde of upper limbs
- Rolling
- Response to auditory stimulus
- Recognition of mother and surroundings
- Irritability of the child

Prone Observation

- Attitude at arrest

- Weight bearing
- Head holding in midline
- Pelvic status
- Mode of ambulation
- Other factors to be examined:

S. no.	Factor	Value
1.	Height of the baby	50 cm
2.	Head circumference	34–35 cm
3.	Chest circumference	Usually 3–4 cm less than head circumference
4.	Respiratory status	30–40/min
5.	Heart rate	120–140 beats/min
6.	Birth weight	2.5–3.5 kg

On Examination

Reflex Maturation

Reflex	Normal age	Status (present/absent)
Neonatal Reflexes		
Dolls eye	Birth–10 days	
Rooting, sucking and swallowing	Birth–3–4 months	
Palmar grasp and plantar grasp	Birth–3–4 months	
Placing reactions	Birth–6 months	
Moros reflex	Birth–3–4 months	
Automatic standing and walking	Birth–1½ months	
Galants reflex	6 months	

Contd.

Contd.

Spinal Reflexes		Labyrinthine righting	2–6 months
Flexor withdrawl reflex	Birth–2 months	Body rightning on head	6 months–4–5 years
Extensor thrust	Birth–2 months	Body rightning on body	6 months–4–5 years
Crossed extensor	Birth–2 months		
Brainstem reflexes		Parachute reactions	6 months
ATNR	Birth–3–4 months	Cortical reactions–equilibrium	—
STNR	Birth–3–4 months	Prone	6 months
Tonic labyrinthine	Birth–3–4 months	Supine	8 months
Positive supporting reaction	Birth–6 months	Quadruped	8–10 months
		Sitting	8–10 months
Midbrain Reaction		Kneeling	15 months
Neck righting	Birth–6 months	Standing	15 months

Motor Examination

- Tone
- Grading on modified Ashworth scale:
- Voluntary control/MMT (power):

	Flexion	Extension	Adduction	Abduction	Medial rotation	Lateral rotation
Shoulder						
Elbow						
Wrist						
Hip						
Knee						
Ankle						
Cervical						
Lumbar						

Modify the movement names as per the joints

Range of Motion

	Flexion		Extension		Adduction		Abduction		Medial rotation		Lateral rotation	
	A	P	A	P	A	P	A	P	A	P	A	P
Shoulder												
Elbow												
Wrist												
Hip												
Knee												
Ankle												
Cervical												
Lumbar												

Modify the names of the movements as per joint when applicable
A–active range of motion   P–passive range of motion

Musculoskeletal Assessment

- Tightness/contracture/deformity
- Limb length and limb girth

HIGHER FUNCTION

Level of Consciousness

Glasgow Coma Scale

- Eye opening 4.
  - ↳ None—even to pain
  - ↳ To pain—pain from stimulus to limbs
  - ↳ To speech—opens eyes on verbal approach
  - ↳ Spontaneous—opens eye spontaneously
- Motor response 6.
  - ↳ None—to any pain, limbs remain flaccid.
  - ↳ Extension to pain—shoulder adducted/internally rotated, forearm pronated.
  - ↳ Abnormal flexion to pain—shoulder flexes/adducts.
  - ↳ Flexion/withdrawal to pain—(flexion of elbow, supination of forearm, flexion of wrist when supraorbital pressure applied; pulls part of the body away when nailbed pinched.
  - ↳ Localizes pain—arm attempts to remove supraorbital pain.
  - ↳ Obeys commands—follows command.
- Verbal response 5.
  - ↳ None—as stated
  - ↳ Incomprehensive—moaning but no words
  - ↳ Inappropriate—random or exclamatory articulated speech, but no conversational exchange.
  - ↳ Confused—the patient responds to questions coherently but there is some disorientation and confusion.
  - ↳ Oriented—patient responds coherently and appropriately to questions such as the patient's name and age, where they are and why, the year, month, etc.)

Scoring

Eye opening	4
Motor response	6
Verbal response	5
Total	**15**

Generally, brain injury is classified as:

- Severe, with GCS ≤8 that is also a generally accepted definition of a coma
- Moderate, with GCS 9–12
- Minor, with GCS ≥13.

Memory

1. Instant
2. Short term
3. Long term

Intelligence: Checked by simple mathematical calculations.

Behavior:

Orientation:

1. By place
2. By time
3. By person

Speech: Identify for any speech disorder related to neurological imbalance.

CRANIAL NERVE ASSESSMENT

Sensory Assessment

Superficial

- Pain
- Touch
  - ↳ Fine
  - ↳ Crude
- Temperature

Deep

- Pressure
- Vibrations
- Joint position sense
- Joint kinesthetic sense

Combined Cortical Sensation

- Tactile localization
- Stereognosis (object recognition)
- Two-point discrimination
- Coordination and balance

FUNCTIONAL EVALUATION

HISTORY OF MILESTONE DEVELOPMENT

Pediatric Assessment

HISTORY FROM MOTHER

Take the prenatal, natal and post natal hisotry from the mother and identify any causes.

Prenatal	• TORCH infections [toxoplasmosis, rubella, cytomegalovirus, herpes simplex virus • Smoking/alcoholism • Diabetes/hypertension • Fall • Consanginous marriages • Rh incompatibily • Drug addicted mother
Perinatal	• Forceps delivery • Breech presentation • Premature delivery • Entangling of placenta around the neck
Postnatal	• Jaundice • Fall from height • Neonatal infections, e.g. meningitis

Take the Apgar score history from the case file.

APGAR SCORING

It is a quantitative method for assessing infants respiratory, circulatory, and neurological status immediately after the birth.

• *Timing:* 1 min, 5 min, 10–20 min after the birth.

Score	Effect
8–10	Normal
5–7	Moderate asphyxia
Less than 4	Severe distress

S. no.	Factor	Score=0	Score=1	Score = 2
1.	Heart rate	Absent	Less than 100 beats/min	More than 100 beats/min
2.	Respiratory effort	Absent	Slow, irregular cry	Good cry
3.	Muscle tone	Limp	Some flexion in extremities	Active good flexor tone

Contd.

S. no.	Factor	Score=0	Score=1	Score = 2
4.	Response to catheter	No response	Grimace	Cough/sneeze
5.	Colour of baby	Blue/Raif	Body pink and extremities blue	Completely pink

• As in newborn, extremities are always blue immediately after birth, ideal score is never 10 at 1 min but 9.

Check for the associated symptoms:

• Mental retardation
• Convulsions
• Visual deficits
• Hearing defects
• Perceptual problems
• Learning disabilities
• Feeding problem
• Emotional and behavioural problems
• Speech and language disorders

ON OBSERVATION

Observe for any dysmorphic features of the child:

• Low set eyes and ears
• Frontal bossing
• Delayed closure of anterior fontanelle
• Cleft lip/cleft palate
• Excessive drooling of saliva
• Irregular dentition

Other factors to be assessed:

S. no.	Effect	Value
1	Height of the baby	50 cm
2.	Head circumference	34–35 cm
3.	Chest circumference	Usually 3–4 cm less than head circumference
4.	Respiratory status	30–40 min
5.	Heart rate	120–140 beats/min
6.	Birth weight	2.5–3.5 kg

Supine Observation

Observe the baby and note the features under the following headings:

- Attitutde at rest
- Symmetry of the body
- Involuntary movements
- Position of the head
- Visual fixation and tracking
- Attitude of upper limbs
- Rolling
- Response to auditory stimulus
- Recognition of mother and surroundings
- Irritability of the child

Prone Observation

- Attitude at rest
- Weight bearing
- Head holding in midline
- Pelvic status
- Mode of ambulation

ILLINGWORTH SCALE

- Along with birth asphyxia, preterm babies also form a major group in cerebral palsy children.
- Therefore, a preterm infant should be identified from normal term infant.
- Illingworth scale differentiates a preterm baby [risk baby] from full term baby.

There are 14 factors present in the scale

S. no.	Factor	Preterm	Full term
1	Sleep	Disturbed small sleep cycles	Sound sleep
2.	Movements	Faster/bizzare/uncoordinated	Coordinated
3.	Cry	Cry is frequent/feeble/not prolonged	Prolonged vigorous cry
4.	Feeding behaviour	Cannot relied upon to demand feeds may be unable to suck and swallow regurgitation—cyanotic attacks	Can be relied upon for feeds rooting/sucking/swallowing-normal
5.	Muscle tone	Less flexor tone	Good flexor tone
6.	Posture of baby	*Prone:* Flat pelvis and knees at the side of abdomen Acute flexion at hips	*Prone:* Pelvis high knees draw up under abdomen

Contd.

S. no.	Factor	Preterm	Full term
		Supine: Lower limbs externally rotated and ab-ducted. Head turned to one side	*Supine:* Limbs are strongly flexed, head aligned to trunk
7.	Head rotation	Head can be rotated so far that chin is well beyond acromion	Chin can be rotated only as far as acromion
8.	Scarf sign	Hand reaches beyond opposite acromion	Hand doesn't go beyond opposite acromion
9.	Wrist flexion	Wrist flexion is incomplete. There is a window between hand and forearm.	Complete wrist flexion. No gap between palm and forearm.
10.	Grasp	Less than 28 weeks, it is weak	Strong palmar grasp
11.	Knee extension	When hip is flexed completely knee can be fully extended	After complete hip flexion, knee extension is short of 20 degrees
12.	Dorsiflexion of foot	Dorsiflexion of foot is incomplete	Complete dorsiflexion such that the dorsum of foot touches shin of tibia
13.	Automatic walking	28 weeks—feeble 32 weeks—walks on toes 40 weeks—walks with foot flat	Normal walk
14.	Horizontal suspension	Hangs limply no flexion of limbs	Flexes upper and lower limbs strongly

VOJTA'S REACTIONS

These are useful for diagnosis of brain damage in infants.

Dr. Vojta, a German pediatric neurologist, standardized 7 postural reflexes along with neurological and behavioral assessment technique to diagnose the development of cerebral palsy in the neonate.

The 7 reactions are as follows:

• Traction
• Landau
• Axillary suspension
• Vojta's side tilt reaction
• Colli's horizontal suspension
• Pieper and Isbert's reaction
• Colli's vertical suspension reaction

These reactions' development depends on the age of infant from 0–12 months.

Abnormal postural reactions indicate: *"disturbed central coordination" [DCC]*.

The development of cerebral palsy depends upon the severity of DCC.

It is scaled as follows:

Mild DCC	→	3 or less than 3 abnormal reactions
Moderate DCC	→	4–5 abnormal reactions
Severe DCC	→	6–7 abnormal reactions

S. no.	Reac-tion	Elicitation and body part to be observed	Normal response
1.	Traction	Infant is slowly pulled up from supine to an angle of 45 degrees. Head and lower limbs are observed	Complete head lag, but head does not fall on one side. Head remains in center lower limbs in mild flexion
2.	Landau	Prone infant is held in horizontal suspenstion. Head, spine, upper and lower limbs are observed	Head hangs in center. Spine, upper and lower limbs are in flexion

Contd.

S. no.	Reac-tion	Elicitation and body part to be observed	Normal response
3.	Axillary suspen-sion	Infant is lifted in vertical suspension holding just below the axilla Lower limbs are to be observed	Mildly flexed
4.	Vojta's side tilt	Vertically held infant suddenly tiltered to lateral horizontal position. Overlying upper and lower limbs are to be observed.	Overlying upper extremity Moro-Response Lower limb flexed
6.	Pieper and Isbert's vertical suspen-sion	The infant is held by its thighs and lifted suddenly head down in vertical position. Head, spine and upper limb are observed	Head hangs in the center Upper limb—Moro response No response in spine
07.	Colli's vertical suspen-sion reaction	Infant is lifted up with one thigh, head down free lower limb to be observed	Flexion of lower limb

Reflex Maturation

• A reflex is a stereotyped response to a stimulus
• Reflex testing is required for:
  ✎ Early intervention.
  ✎ Level of function identification.
  ✎ Treatment planning.

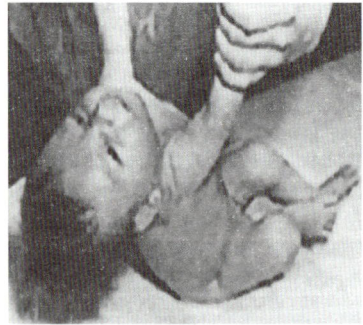

Traction response

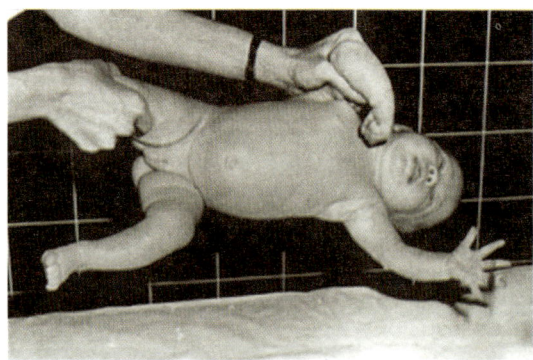

Colli's horizontal suspension

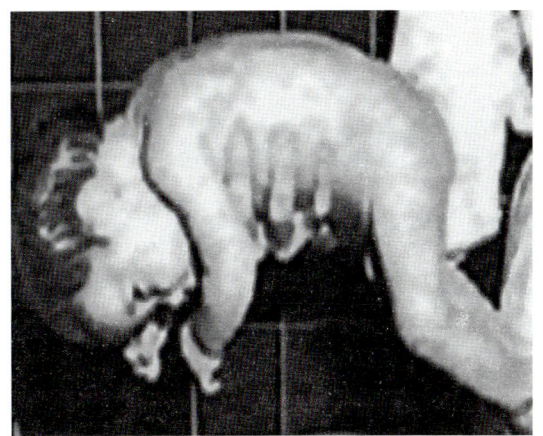

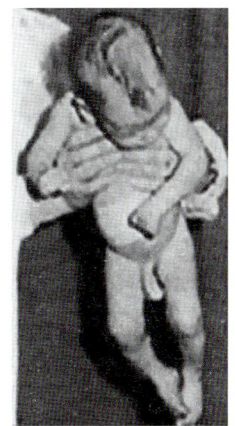

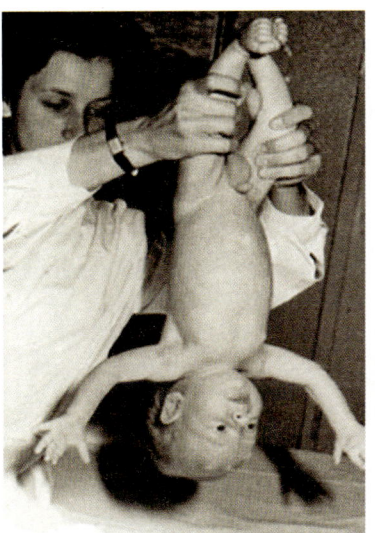

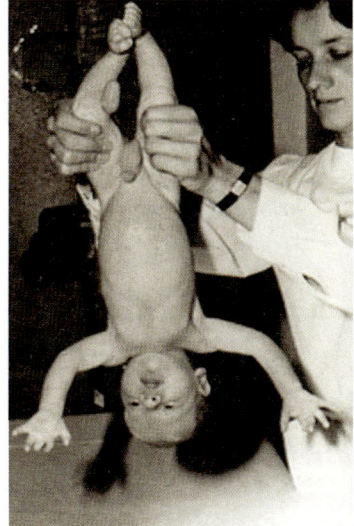

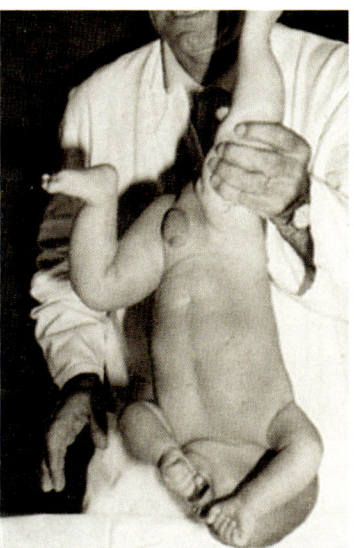

Pieper and Isbert reaction

Colli's vertical suspension

NEONATAL REFLEXES

S. no.	Reflex	Age of normal presence	Stimulus	Response
1.	Doll's eye reflex	Birth–10 days	Baby head is turned to one side	Eyes lag behind.
2.	Rooting reflex	Birth–3–4 months	Light touch around lips	Turning of head, lower lip and tongue on the side of stimulus.
3.	Sucking reflex and swallowing	Birth–3–4 months	Place a finger on baby's lip	Sucking movement of lips and swallows.
4.	Palmar grasp reflex	Birth–4 months	Pressure on palm of hand from ulnar side	Finger flexion with strong grip that persists and resists removal of stimulus.

Contd.

S. no.	Reflex	Age of normal presence	Stimulus	Response
5.	Plantar grasp	Birth–10-11 months	Strong pressure on ball foot	Flexion of toes.
6.	Placing of upper extremity	Birth–6 months	Brush the dorsum of one of baby's hands against edge of the table	Flexion of upper limb with placement of hand on the table.
7.	Placing of lower extremity	Birth–1½ months	Brush the dorsum of the foot against the under edge of the table.	Flexion of the lower limb with placement of foot on the table top.
8.	Moro's reflex	Birth–3–4 days	Dropping the baby head backwards from semi-sitting position	Abduction, external rotation, extension of arms and extension of fingers followed by adduction of arm to midline.
9.	Automatic standing and walking	Birth–1½ months	Place the baby in the vertical suspension near to supporting surface and touch the feet to the ground	Extension of lower limbs as if baby is standing. If pelvis is rotated forwards then child will automatically put steps forward.
10.	Gallant's reflex	Birth–3–6 months	In horizontal suspension, stroke unilateral lumbar region with blunt object	Lateral flexion of trunk on the same side

Spinal Level Reflexes

S. no.	Reflex	Age of normal presence	Stimulus	Response
1.	Flexor withdrawl	Birth–2 months	Quick tactile stimulus applied to the sole of the foot.	Uncontrolled flexion of hip and knee.
2.	Extensor thrust	Birth–2 months	One leg in extension and other fully flexion. Apply pressure on the ball of the foot of flexed leg.	Uncontrolled extension of same leg.
3.	Crossed extensor	Birth–2 months	One leg in flexion and other in extension. Give pressure on the ball of the foot of extended without allowing flexion of the same leg.	The fixed leg extends.

Brainstem Reflexes

S. No.	Reflex	Age of normal presence	Stimulus	Response
1.	Asymmetric tonic neck refex (ATNR)	Birth–4 months	Passively turn the head to 90°	Increase in the extensor tone on face side and increase in flexor tone of limbs on occipital side
2.	Symmetrical tonic neck reflex (STNR)	Birth–4–5 months	Sti 1: Flex the child head bringing his chin towards chest Sti 2: Extension of baby's head	Res1: Flexion of upper extremities and extension of lower extremities Res2: Extension of upper extremities and flexion of lower extremities
3.	Tonic labyrinthine reflex	Birth–3–4 months	Patient in supine and prone position	Increase in flexor tone in prone position and extensor tone in supine

Contd.

S. No.	Reflex	Age of normal presence	Stimulus	Response
4.	Positive supporting reactions	Birth–6 months	Patient upright standing firm contact on ball of foot to floor	Rigid extension of lower limbs resulting from co-contraction of flexors and extensors

Midbrain Reactions

S. No.	Reflex	Age of normal presence	Stimulus	Response
1.	Neck righting reflex	Birth–3 months	In supine position, turn the baby's head to one side and hold it in that position	Body rotates on the same side as a whole (log rolling)
2.	Labyrinthine righting	2 months–lifelong	Baby is blind folded, suspended in space by holding at pelvis. The baby is tipped sideways so that head is laterally flexed	Head brought into horizontal position
3.	Body righting on head	6 months–5 years	Baby is blind folded and first placed in supine then in prone	The head is brought back to vertical position
4.	Body on body righting	6 months–4–5 years	Baby in supine, passively turn the head to one side	Segmental rolling on turned side
5.	Parachute reaction	6 months–lifelong	Baby is held in prone suspension at pelvis, push baby to the side with sufficient surprise and force that he/she believes his head will contact the supporting surface	Extension of all the four limbs

CORTICAL REACTIONS

Equilibrium is tested on equilibrium board in all the functional positions or by pushing the baby from static posture.

S. no.	Equilibrium	Age attained
1.	Prone	6 months
2.	Supine	8 months
3.	Quadriped	8–10 months
4.	Sitting	8–10 months
5.	Kneeling	15 months
6.	Standing	15–18 months

DEVELOPMENT OF MILESTONES

Try to record the age at which a milestone is obtained from the mother or the caretaker. Milestone development is very important tool for identifying the risk babies from full term babies.

Development is a concept which implies both growth and maturation.

Definition: Growth is not just an increase in size but the development increasingly more complex interconnections within the brain.

Principles of Normal Development

1. Development is a continuous process, rate of development in each field is different though sequence is same.
2. Development is related to maturation of nervous system which is cephalocaudal in direction and proximal to distal.
3. General mass activity is replaced by specific individual response.
4. Primitive reflexes should be lost before the corresponding voluntary control is achieved.
5. At first, brainstem, thalamus and basal ganglia are dominent in development. The rapid growth of cerebral cortex and cerebellum taking place later.
6. The blood supply during development from subependymal plate to the cerebral cortex. During 3rd trimester, circulation shifts from central to cortical and white matter orientation.
7. Early development is directed towards decrease of flexor tone.

Note: In full term newborn baby, there is pre-dominance of extensor tone in neck and flexor tone in limbs.

Prone Development

Attitude at Birth

Reflexes present are:
 a. Neonatal and spinal
 b. Positive supporting
 c. Neck righting

At 1–3 Months

Reflexes present are:
1. Labyrinthine
2. Righting.

At 3 Months

1. ATNR—decreased
2. STNR—increased
3. Galant's reflex—decreases.

At 6 Months

1. Palmar grasp integrates.
2. Chest off the supporting surface.
3. Weight-bearing on open hands.
4. Visual flied improved.

At 7–10 Months

1. Learns equilibrium and weight
2. Walks sideways with support

At 12 Months

1. Confident to walk forward
2. Keeps hands out in abduction
3. Broad "BOS" (base of support)
4. Few steps alone possible.
5. Walks if held by hands.

Supine Development

At Birth

1. Doll's eye—positive
2. Pelvis—off the support.
3. Rooting, sucking, swallowing—positive
4. Weight-bearing on head and upper trunk.

At 3rd Month

1. Trunk flat on support.
2. Hands come to midline.
3. Eye–hand regard positive.

At 4th Month

Isolated arm movements.

At 4½–5 Months

1. Able to take hands across midline.
2. Segmented, rolling.

At 6th Month

1. Child becomes aware of his body parts.
2. Good hip flexion and extension.
3. Transfer of objects from one hand to other hand. Palmar grasp integrates.
4. Parachute reaction absent.

At 7th Month

1. Eye–hand–foot coordination.
2. Developments of parachute reactions.
    a. Forward—7 months
    b. Sideways—8 months
    c. Backwards—9 months.

23

Cardiorespiratory Assessment

Cardiopulmonary Assessment Form

SUBJECTIVE ASSESSMENT   DOA: ....

Name: .... Age: .... Sex: .... Marital status: ....

Socioeconomic status:... Occupation: ....

Address: ....

....

Chief Complaint

History: ....

....

Present History: ....

....

Past History: ....

....

Personel History: ....

....

Family History: ....

....

Medical History: ....

....

Medication History: ....

....

OBJECTIVE ASSESSMENT

On observation:
General appearence of the patient:
Built of the patient:
Level of awareness:
Color of the skin:
Facial signs or expressions:
Demusset's sign:
Jugular vein engorgement:
Hypertrophy of accessory muscles of respiration
Breathing pattern
Swelling:
Scars:
Clubbing of digits:

On Palpation

Temperature:
Tenderness:
Tracheal/mediastinal shift:
Vocal fremitus:

Distal Pulses

Distal pulse	Rate	Rhythm	Cha-racter	Symmetry Right	Left
Carotid					
Axillary					
Brachial					
Radial					
Femoral					
Tibial					
Dorsipedis					

Edema:
Temperature:
Blood pressure:
Sbp:
Dbp:
Pulse pressure:
Mean BP:
Casual BP:
Basal BP:

JUGULAR VENOUS PRESSURE

Procedure: Ask them to turn their head to look away from you. Look across the neck between the two heads of sternocleidomastoid for a pulsation. If you do see a pulsation, you need to determine whether it is the JVP— if it is,

then the pulsation is non-palpable, obliterable by compressing distal to it, and will be exaggerated by performing the hepatojugular reflex.

Having warned the patient that it may cause some discomfort, press down on the liver. This will cause the JVP to rise further. If you decide the pulsation is due to the JVP, note its vertical height above the sternal angle.

APEX HEART BEAT

On Examination

Analysis of Chest Shape and Dimensions

Anteroposterior diameter	Lateral diameter
Result	

Posture Analysis of the Patient

Determinant	Result
Posture preferred by the patient	
Level of shoulders	
Vertebral curves	
Chest shape	
Relaxing postures adopted	

Examination of Breathing Pattern

Determinant	Result
Rate	
Regularity	
Pattern	
Abnormal breathing (if any)	
If dyspnoea present, then grade of dyspnoea.	

Examination of Chest Mobility

Determinant	Result
Upper lobe expansion	
Middle lobe expansion	
Lower lobe expansion	

Examination of Extent of Excursion

Determinant	Inspiration (in inches)	Expiration (in inches)
Axilla		
Xiphoid		
Lower costal		

On Percussion

Determinant	Right anterior	Right posterior	Left anterior	Left posterior
Result				

On Auscultation

Normal Breath Sounds

Breath sounds	Description	Result
Vesicular	Soft, low-pitched, breezy heard over the most of the chest except at the trachea and between the scapulae, they are audible longer on inspiration	
Bronchial	Loud, hollow or tubular high-pitched sounds heard over the main stem bronchi and trachea. They are heard equally on inspiration and expiration, a slight pause is present between inspiration and expiration	
Broncho-vesicular	Softer than bronchial breath sounds equally heard on inspiration and expiration, but there is no pause. The sounds are heard in the supraclavicular, suprascapular and parasternal anteriorly and between the scapulae posteriorly	
Tracheal	Heard on trachea	

Adventitious Breath Sounds

Sound	Right	Left
Crackles / rales		
Wheezes / rhonchi		

HEART MURMURS

- *Grade 1*: Murmur is barely audible with special effort.
- *Grade 2*: Murmur is faint but easily heard.
- *Grade 3*: Murmur is moderately loud.
- *Grade 4*: Murmur is very loud, there may be a thrill.
- *Grade 5*: Murmur is extremely loud, but one edge of the stethscope must be on the chest to hear.
- *Grade 6*: Murmur is exceptionally loud and is audible with the stethoscope just above the chest.

Normal Heart Sounds

Heart sound	Description	Result
S1	Best heard at lower sternal border and apex of heart. Increased sound is heard in mitral stenosis, tachycardia. Decreased sound in fibrotic or calcified mitral valve, severe LV dysfunction, mitral regurgitation.	
S2	Heard loudest at aortic and pulmonary areas often split in to two components A2 (aortic) P2 (pulmonary) with increased spilitting on inspiration and decreased splitting on expiration. Increased A2 is heard in hypertension, congenital defects, transposition of great vessels. Decreased A2 in aortic stenosis. Increased P2 in pulmonary hypertension, thin chested individuals. Decreased P2 in pulmonary stenosis.	
S3 (Ventricular gallop)	A low-pitched heart sound heard with patient lying on the left side so the apex of the heart is close to the chest wall. This is physiologic in individuals below 40 years of age Commonly heard in impaired LV function, congenital heart diseases. Valvular diseases, systemic or pulmonary hypertension, pericarditis, severe anemia, thyrotoxicosis, pregnancy.	
S4 (Atrial gallop)	A low-pitched sound heard in late diastole Commonly heard in LV or RV hypertrophy, arrhythmias.	

EXAMINATION OF COUGH

Determinant	Result
Strength	
Length	
Frequency	
Type (productive/non-productive)	

SPUTUM ANALYSIS

Determinent	Result
Colour	
Consistency	
Amount (voloume)	
Odour (smell)	

RANGE OF MOTION

Joint/movement	Left	Right
Shoulder		
Flexion		
Extension		
Adduction		

Contd.

Joint/movement	Left	Right
Abduction		
Medial rotation		
Lateral rotation		
Neck		
Flexion		
Lateral flexion		
Extension		
Rotation		

MUSCLE POWER

ENDURANCE TESTS

PSYCHOLOGICAL ASSESSMENT:

INVESTIGATIONS:

PROBLEM LISTING:

PHYSIOTHERAPY MANAGEMENT:

Observation Skills in Cardiopulmonary Cases

GENERAL APPEARANCE OF THE PATIENT

Describe how the patient looks on observation.

Built of the Patient

Describe the body type of the patient, grade the patient as normal, obese or cachectic.

Before you describe, you need to know the BMI of the patient (body mass index) (please refer BMI assessment).

Level of Awareness

Describe whether the patient is alert, responsive, cooperative, lethargic, disoriented or inattentive.

Color of the Skin

Check whether there is any color change in the skin, e.g. cyanosis (bluish discoloration of the skin)

- *Malar flush*: Long-standing MS, rash across the nose and nose in SLE.
- Brick red color of polycythemia (may cause HTN, thrombosis, MI).
- Bronze skin in hemochromatosis (cardio-myopathy).
- Pale skin seen in anemia.
- Brown + buccal pigmentation in Addison's disease (hypotension).
- Flushing and telangiectasia in carcinoid syndrome (tricuspid and pulmonary valve disease).
- Moon face in Cushing's disease (HTN).
- Coarseness and dryness in myxedema (brady-cardia, heart failure, PE).
- Cyanosis (bluish discoloration of the skin).

TYPES OF CYANOSIS

1. *Central cyanosis:* Blue tongue, lips, and extremities with warm peripheries (CHD, lung disease as emphysema, pneumonia, ARDS, chronic bronchitis, sometimes CHF).
2. *Peripheral cyanosis* (result from sluggish circulation in the peripheries) reduction in oxygenated Hb occur in capillaries (extremities are blue and cold)
   Etiologies: Low CO, hypovolemic shock.
3. *Differential cyanosis* (lower limb cyanosed, upper limb pink) in CHD: PDA with revered shunt due to PHTN.
4. *Reversed differential cyanosis.* The cyanosis of the fingers exceeds that of the toes; seen in transposition of the great vessels (blood from

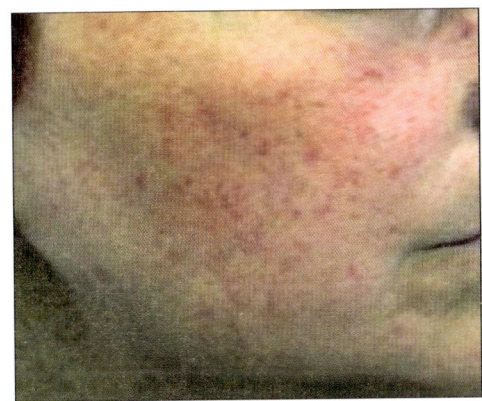

Hemochromatosis

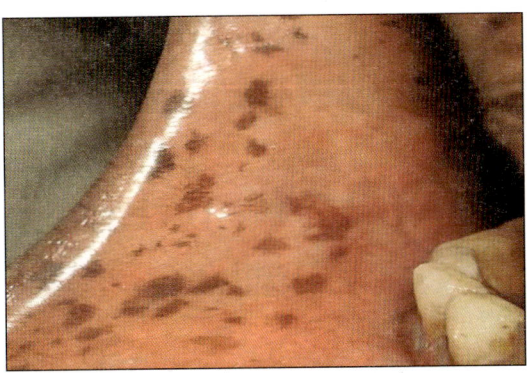

Buccal pigmentation

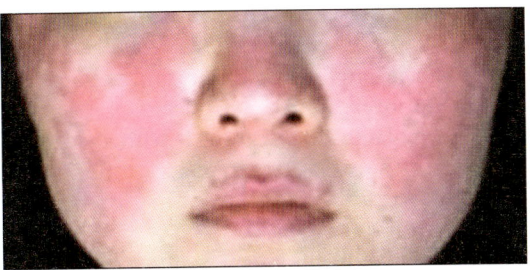

Malar flush

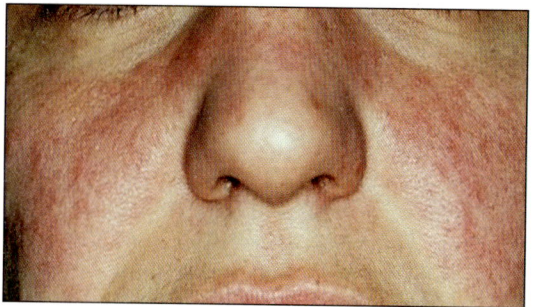

Polycythemia

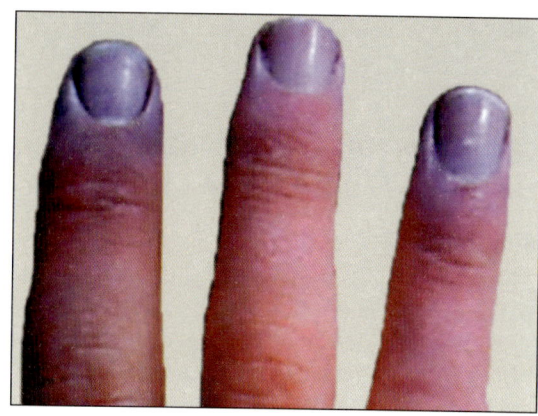

Peripheral cyanosis

RV ejected into the AO reaches the upper limbs and head, blood from LV ejected into PA reaches the lower limb via PDA.

FACIAL SIGNS OR EXPRESSIONS

Check the following and interpret.

Observation	Inference
Focused or dilated pupils: Argyll-Robertson pupil (pupil react to accommodation not to the light)	Atrial regurgitation, calcification in the ascending aorta
Nasal flaring	Signs of respiratory distress
Profused sweating	Myocardial infarction, coronary artery disease
Distressed appearance	Chest discomfort in angina,
Xanthelasma	Hypercholesterolemia, diabetes mellitus
Lid edema	Endocrinal disorder (myxedema)
Exophthalmos	Thyrotoxicosis
Corneal arcus	In young people, it indicates severe hypercholesterolemia
Blue sclera	Atrial regurgitation, atrial septal defect
Osler's nodules (0.5–1 cm painful reddish-brown subcutaneous papules occur on the tips of the fingers or toes, palm of the hand, plantar aspect of the feet	Bacterial endocarditis

Demusset's Sign

The head nods in time with the heartbeat—seen rarely in severe aortic regurgitation.

Jugular Vein Engorgement

Visualize the jugular venous pulse with the patient supine and the head and neck on the pillows at a 45° angle.

Report

Observation	Inference
Normal	Normal
Bilateral distension	Congestive cardiac failure / right side heart failure

HYPERTROPHY OF ACCESSORY MUSCLES OF RESPIRATION

Observe the hypertrophy of the accessory muscles of respiration like trapezius, sternocleidomastoid, pectorals, scaleni. It is observed in patients with early chronic lung diseases and weakness of diaphragm.

BREATHING PATTERN

Observe the patient breathing and report.
Normal breathing is as follows:
- Normal relaxed breathing is with abdominal rise by symmetric expansion of the lateral ribs without use of accessory muscles of respiration.
- Normal expiration is passive expiration.

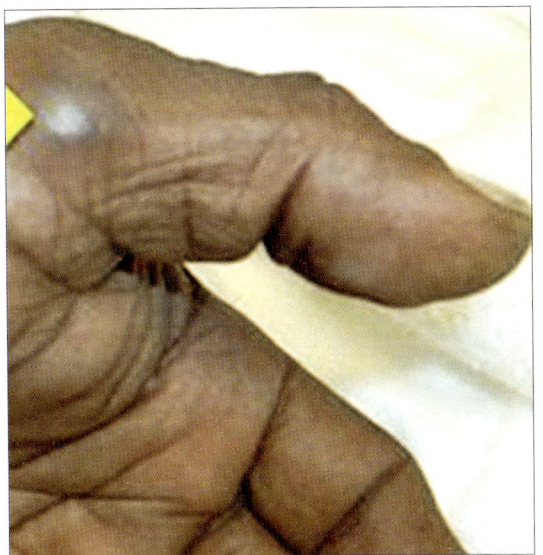

Osler's nodules

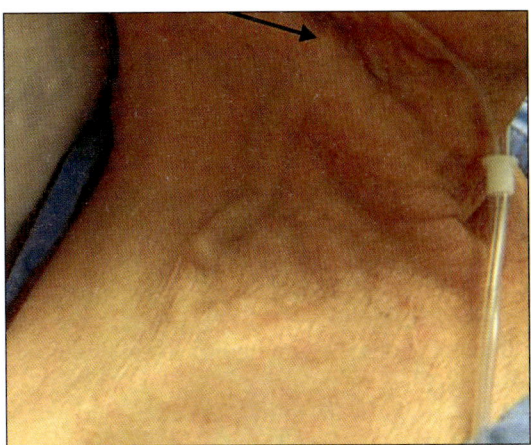

Distended jugular vein

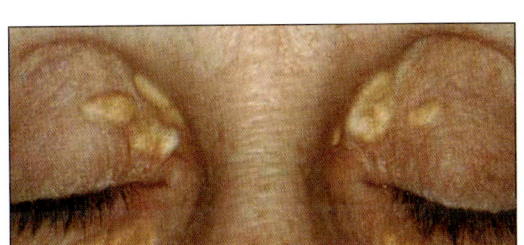

Xanthelasma

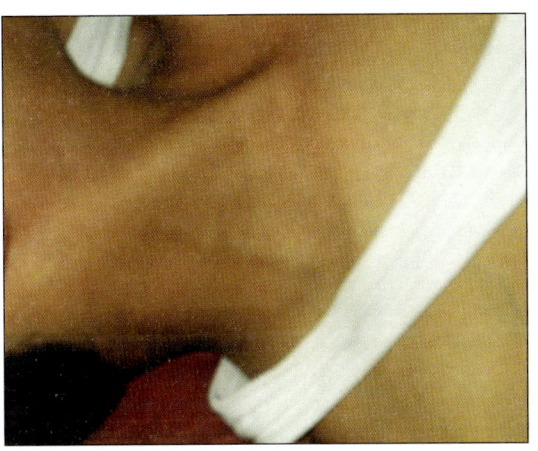

Normal jugular vein

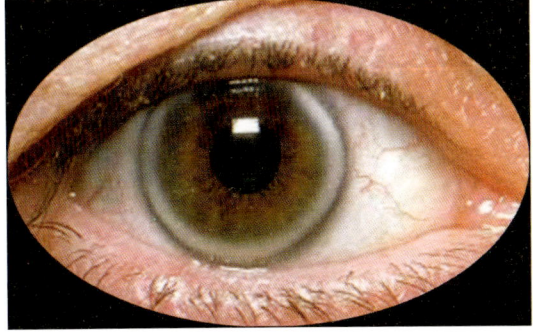

Corneal arcus

Observation	Result
Supraclavicular or intercostal retractions occurring with inspiration	Labored breathing seen in COPD
Use of pursed lip breathing	Indicates difficulty with expiration often seen in patients with COPD
Use of accessory muscles of respiration	Pulmonary edema, asthma, pneumonia

Contd.

Observation	Result
Breathlessness + wheezing	Asthma, left ventricular failure
Stridor	It indicates upper airway obstruction and is a life-threatening situation
Chyne-Stokes respiration	Congestive heart failure, over sedation

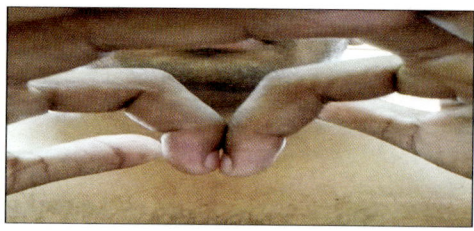

Schamroth's test

Clubbing of Digits

Obliteration of the nail bed angle is known as clubbing.

Procedure: Schamroth's test or Schamroth's window test (originally demonstrated by South African cardiologist Leo Schamroth on himself) is a popular test for clubbing. When the distal phalanges (bones nearest the fingertips) of corresponding fingers of opposite hands are directly opposed (place fingernails of same finger on opposite hands against each other, nail to nail), a small diamond-shaped "window" is normally apparent between the nail beds. If this window is obliterated, the test is positive and clubbing is present.

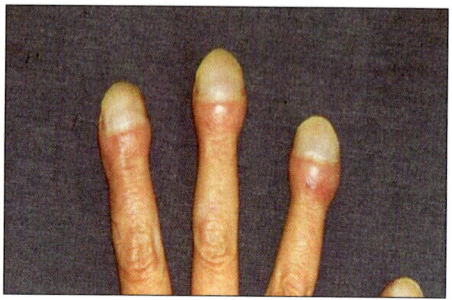

Drumstick-like fingers

Grade	Description
1	Softening of the nail beds.
2	Obliteration of the nail bed angle.
3	Parrot beak appearance of the fingers.
4	Drumstick-like fingers.

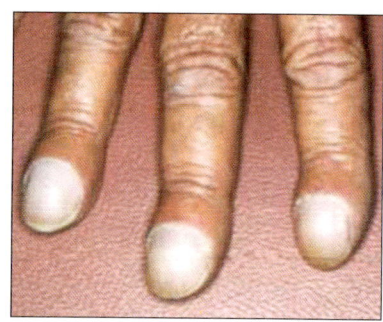

Parrot beak appearance

On Palpation in Cardiopulmonary Cases

TEMPERATURE

Rise of temperature indicates acute infection or inflammation.

Tenderness

All the accessory muscles of respiration are palpated and checked whether there is tenderness or not.

Tenderness is graded as follows:

Grade	Description
Severe	Patient shows grimace on the face with touch.
Moderate	Patient shows grimace on the face on holding.
Mild	Patient shows grimace on the face on pressing the muscle.
Absent	No tenderness.

Edema

Technique for evaluation of edema:
1. Examiner impresses thumb on to the skin over bony surface
   (a) Tibia   (b) Fibula   (c) Sacrum
2. Withdraw thumb
3. Measure depth of pit and record in millimeters check for the edema and report it as follows:
   ↳ *Location of edema*: Precisely locate the anatomical position of the edema, e.g. *a localized edema on the dorsum of right forearm.*
   ↳ *Indurated or non-indurated:* Indurated edema will be hard and firm and non-movable, i.e. it will not be able to drain physically by maneuvers like Effleurage.

- Non-indurated edema will be movable and could be drained by physical maneuvers like Effleurage.
- Indurated edema can be due to local trauma, inflammation or infection.
- It can be seen bilaterally in cases of heart diseases, renal dysfunction, abdominal mass, lung dysfunctions.
   ↳ *Pitting or non-pitting*: If there is a observable swelling over the body tissues due to fluid accumulation and when a pressure is applied over the area, if there is an indentation that persists for sometime after the release of pressure it is called pitting edema.
   ↳ It is commonly seen in systemic diseases like hypertension.
   ↳ If there is no indentation seen after the pressure is released, then it is non-pitting.
   ↳ *Localized or generalized*: If there is swelling observed on a precise area, it is localized and if there is a gross swelling, then it is called as generalized.

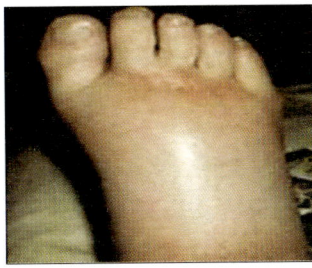

Indurated edema

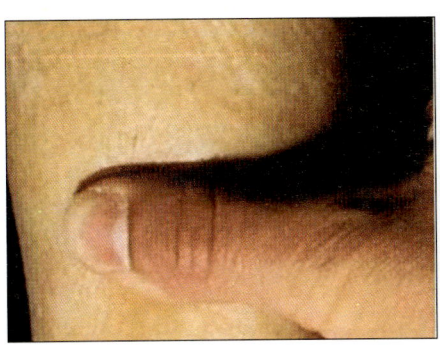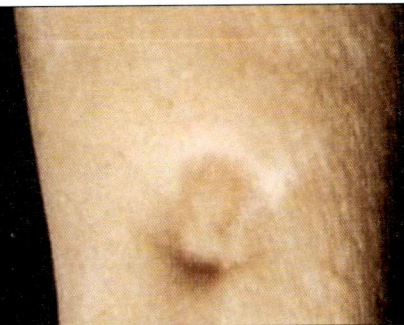

Pitting type edema

Tracheal Shift/Mediastinal Shift

Trachea is normally oriented centrally in relation to the suprasternal notch indicating the symmetry of the mediastinum.

The trachea shifts as a result of asymmetrical intrathoracic pressures or lung volumes.

Procedure: To identify a mediastinal shift:

1. Ask the patient to sit facing you with head in the midline and slightly flex the neck to relax the sternocleidomastoid muscle.
2. With your index finger, gently palpate the soft tissue space on the either side of trachea at the suprasternal notch.
3. Trace the trachea with the index finger and feel the position of the trachea.
4. Determine whether the trachea is palpable in the midline or shifted to one side.

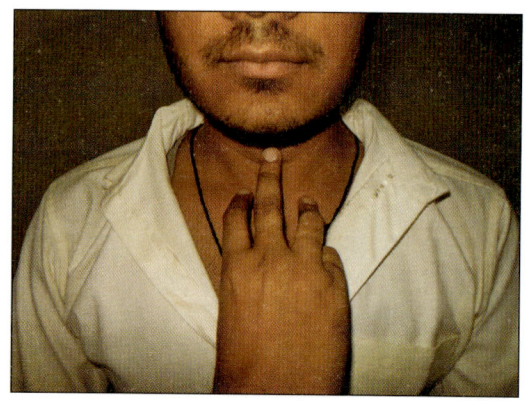

INFERENCE

The position of the trachea shifts as the result of asymmetrical intrathoracic pressures or lung volumes.

The trachea will shift towards the low intrathoracic pressure, e.g. if a patient underwent lobectomy, then the shift will be towards the operated side and if a patient has haemothorax, the shift will be towards opposite side.

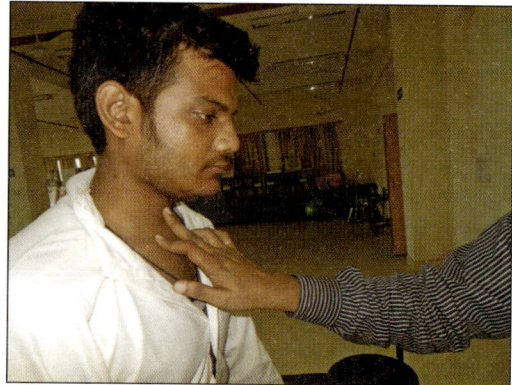

Vocal Fremitus

Vocal or tactile fremitus is the vibration felt while palpating over the chest wall as a patient speaks

Procedure: Vocal or tactile fremitus is the vibration felt while palpating over the chest wall as a patient speaks.

Place your palms lightly over the chest wall and ask the patient to repeat the word '99' several times.

Normally, fremitus is felt uniformly on the chest wall.

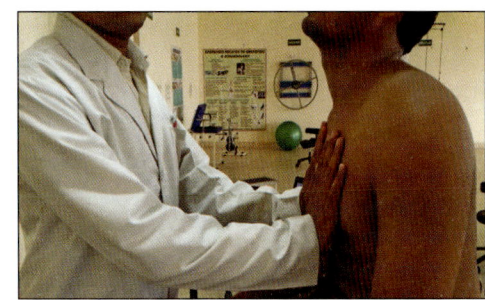

Result

Fremitus	Interpretation
Felt equally and uniformly on the chest areas	Normal
Increased	Secretions in the airways
Decreased or absent	Airway obstruction or air trapped

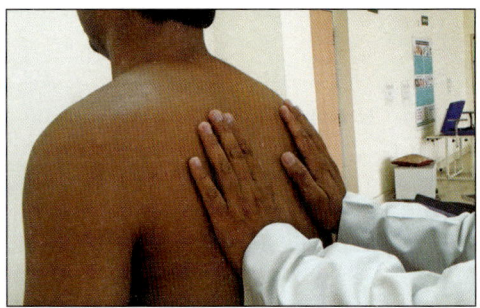

Examination of the Distal Pulses

Examine carotid, axillary, brachial, radial, femoral, tibial and dorsalis pedis pulses.

Systematic Examination of Pulses

Artery	Technique to palpate	Need
1. Radial artery	• Radial side of wrist over the radial tuberosity • With tips of index and middle fingers	• To assess rate and rhythm. • Recorded simultaneously with femoral pulse to detect delay.
2. Brachial artery	• Medial border of humerus at elbow medial to biceps tendon. • Palpate with the thumb of examiner's dominant hand	• To assess the pulse character. • And to confirm rhythm.
3. Carotid artery	• Press examiner's left thumb against patient's larynx. • Press back to feel carotid artery against precervical muscles.	• Checked for pulse character and to judge ventricular function • Useful for identification of carotid stenosis. • Mostly used to check the pulse during the CPR (cardiopulmonary resuscitation)

Contd.

Artery	Technique to palpate	Need
4. Femoral artery	• Patient lying flat and undressed. • Place finger directly above pubic ramus and midway between pubic tubercle and ASIS (anterior superior iliac spine)	• To assess cardiac output. • To detect radiofemoral delay. • To assess the PVD (peripheral vascular disease)
5. Popliteal artery	• Deep within the popliteal fossa. • Compress against posterior of distal femur with knee slightly flexed.	• Mainly to assess peripheral vascular disease in chronic systemic diseases like diabetes to check for vascular disturbances
6. Dorsalis pedis (DP) and tibialis posterior (TP) arteries (foot)	• Lateral to extensor hallucis longus (DP). • Posterior to medial malleolus (TP).	• Same as above.
7. The abdominal aorta	• With the flat of the hand per abdomen, as body habitus allows.	• To assess peripheral vascular disease. • To detect aneurysmal swelling.

Determinant	Inference
Rate	1. Normal rate is 70–100 beats/min *Variations:* 2. Tachycardia is increased in heart rate and is seen in anxiety, pain, congestive cardiac failure, hyperthyroidism, anemia, fever and due to some medications 3. Bradycardia is decreased in heart rate and is seen in myocardial infarction, hyperthyroidism, hypothermia and due to some medications
Rhythm	1. Normal rhythm is sinus rhythm. *Variations:* 2. **Sinus arrhythmia:** There is variation of rate with breathing. It accelerates on inspiration and slows a little on expiration. *Note:* It is commonly seen in the children and young adults but is uncommon over the age of 30. 3. **Pulsus paradoxus:** The pulse slows down on inspiration observed in cases of pericaridal effusion, constrictive pericarditis and severe pneumothorax, bronchial asthma, COPD 4. **Missed or extra beat:** If the pulse is missing by one beat, check whether this is following a regular pattern or irregular pattern . In ventricular failure, a regular pattern in the irregularity is observed. In heart, block can cause an extra beat or missed beat. A random irregularity is a feature of atrial fibrillation.
Character	1. **Collapsing pulse** (water hammer pulse): Jerky pulse with full expansion followed by sudden collapse seen in the cases of atrial regurgitation, persistant ductus arteriosus (PDA) fistulas, pregnancy, Paget's disease, thyrotoxicosis, anemia. 2. **Alternating pulse:** Also known as pulsus alternans (regular rate, amplitude varies from beat to beat) seen in left ventricular failure. 3. **Pulsus bisferiens** (two strong systolic peaks separated by a midsystolic dip): Seen in atrial stenosis. 4. **Anacrotic pulse:** Slow rising pulse. 5. **Diacrotic pulse**: Two systolic and diastolic peaks (sepsis, hypovolemic, cardiogenic shock) 6. **Paradoxic pulse** (amplitude decreases with inspiration and increases during expiration): Seen in cardiac tamponade, COPD, massive PE.
Symmetry	Check whether the pulse is symmetrical on both sides or altered.

Report the pulse in the following format from the observations that are described above.

Distal pulse	Rate	Rhythm	Character	Symmetry	
				Right	Left
Carotid					
Axillary					
Brachial					
Radial					
Femoral					
Tibial					
Dorsalis pedis					

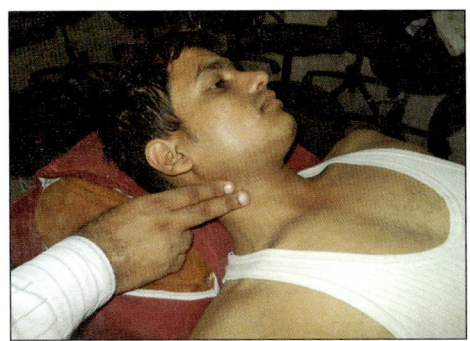

Carotid pulse

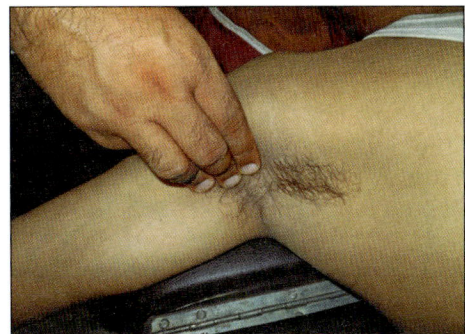

Axillary pulse

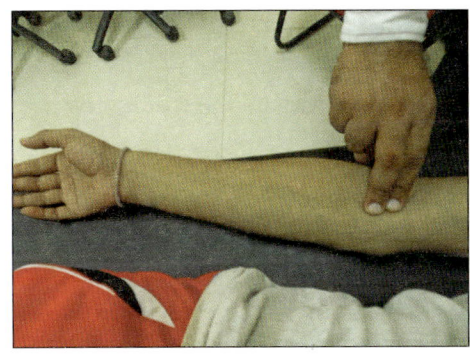

Brachial pulse

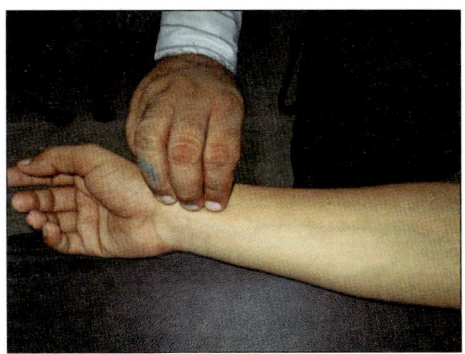

Radial pulse

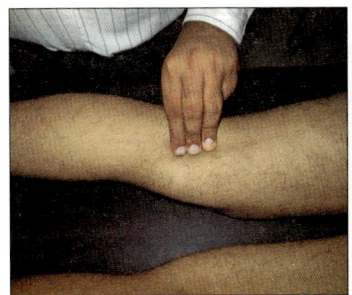

Popliteal pulse

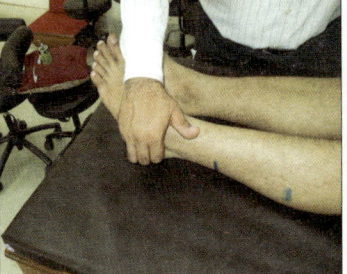

Tibial pulse

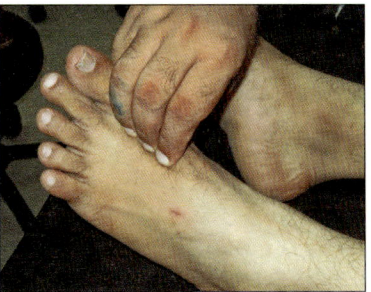

Dorsalis pedis pulse

Recording of Arterial Blood Pressure

It is the lateral pressure exerted by blood on the arterial wall perpendicular to the flow of blood.

Blood pressure is measured by sphygmomanometer.

Systolic blood pressure (SBP): It is the BP during the systole of the heart.

Diastolic blood pressure (DBP): It is the BP during diastole of the heart.

Pulse pressure: It is the difference between systolic and diastolic BP, normal value is 40 mm Hg.

Mean pressure: It is the average pressure in arterial system for entire cardiac cycle.

True mean pressure = diastolic blood pressure +1/3 of pulse pressure

The ratio of SBP, DBP and pulse pressure is 3:2:1.

Casual BP: BP recored during anytime of the day.

Basal BP: It is the BP recorded when the patient is physically and mentally relaxed usually 12 hrs after meal.

> Normal BP is 120/80 mm Hg

PHYSIOLOGICAL VARIATIONS OF THE BP

Age: In the newborn, SBP is 20–60 mm Hg.

After 1 month, it is 90 mm Hg

In adults, it is 120 mm Hg

In old age, it is 150 mm Hg

Sex: In females, BP is 5 to 10 mm Hg less than males.

Diurnal variations: BP is least in the morning. It is 5–10 mm Hg more in the afternoon.

Size: High in obese individuals.

Emotions: SBP increases by 20–30 mm Hg which is due to increased sympathetic activity in emotional excitement.

Sleep: BP falls by 15–20 mm Hg.

Posture: In standing posture, the venous return decreases, cardiac output and SBP decreases by 10–20 mm Hg.

Effect of meals: BP increases due to increased cardiac output after meals.

Exercise: Moderate exercises cause mild increase in cardiac output.

Severe exercise—SBP might increase to 180 mm Hg, DBP decreases to 50 mm Hg.

TECHNIQUE OF MEASURING BLOOD PRESSURE USING SPHYGMOMANOMETER

Apparatus : Stethoscope, sphygmomanometer.

There are two techniques of measuring blood pressure:

- *Palpatory method*—Only SBP can be measured.
- *Auscultatory method*—SBP and DBP can be measured.

Palpatory Method

1. Make the patient sit on a stool infront of you.
2. Ask the patient to relax.
3. Tie the cuff over the cubital fossa firmly.
4. Now feel for the radial pulse.
5. Now inflate the cuff by pressing the bulb until you feel pulselessness.

> When the SBP is higher than 140 mm Hg and DBP higher than 90, it is called as hypertension.
>
> SBP lower than 90 mm Hg and DBP lower than 60 mm Hg then it is called as hypotension.

6. Now slowly deflate the cuff by turning the nozzle.
7. Note the reading where you again start feeling the pulse.
8. The point where the pulse has felt again is the SBP.

> White coat syndrome: It is a condition where the patient BP increases when in hospital or recorded by a doctor and then come back to normal when recorded at home.

Auscultatory Method

1. Make the patient sit on a stool.
2. Ask the patient to relax.
3. Tie the cuff as mentioned above.
4. Now with the help of stethoscope, auscultate the brachial pulse just medial to the biceps tendon in the cubital fossa.
5. Now start inflating the cuff, by pressing the bulb.

6. Inflate until you do not hear the pulse and a complete silence is felt.

7. Inflate a 20 mm Hg further to this point.

8. Now start deflating the cuff, slowly.

9. While deflating, there will be a first tap sound heard, note the reading where you have heard.

10. Followed by tap, there will be continuous murmuring sounds.

11. Note the reading when this murmuring stops.

12. These sounds are called Korotkoff sounds.

13. The point where you have heard the first Tap sound is the SBP and the reading where the murmers stopped is the DBP.

14. Now, report the BP as follows: SBP/DBP mm Hg.

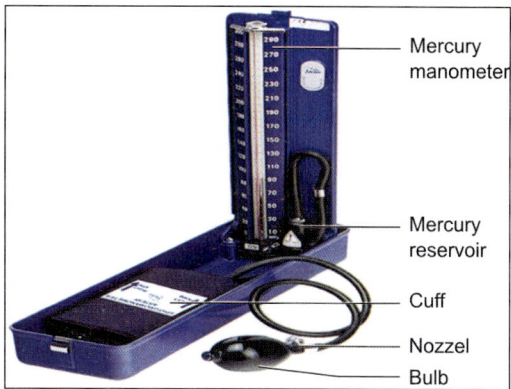

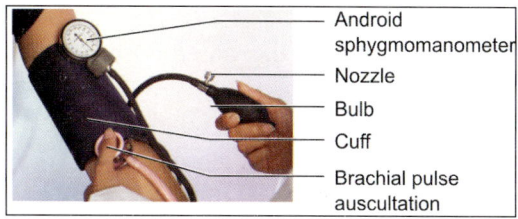

Assessment of Jugular Venous Pressure

JUGULAR VENOUS PRESSURE

Procedure: Ask the patient to turn head to look away from you.

Look across the neck between the two heads of sternocleidomastoid muscle for a pulsation.

If you do see a pulsation, you need to determine whether it is the JVP—if it is then the pulsation is non-palpable, obliterable by compressing distal to it, and will be exaggerated by performing the hepatojugular reflex.

Hepatojugular Reflex

Explain the patient that there will be a bit discomfort in the procedure. Have the consent of the patient.

Make the patient lie in relaxed supine press down on the liver. This will cause the JVP to rise further. If you decide the pulsation is due to the JVP, note its vertical height above the sternal angle.

Using a centimeter ruler, measure the vertical distance between the angle of Louis (manubriosternal joint) and the highest level of jugular vein pulsation.

A straight edge intersecting the ruler at a right angle may be helpful.

Ability to measure jugular venous pressure will be difficult, if pulse is >100 per minute.

In normal individuals, it is usually 3 cm.

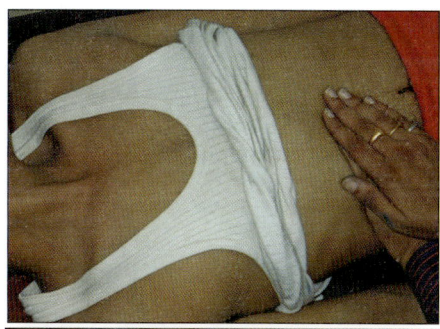

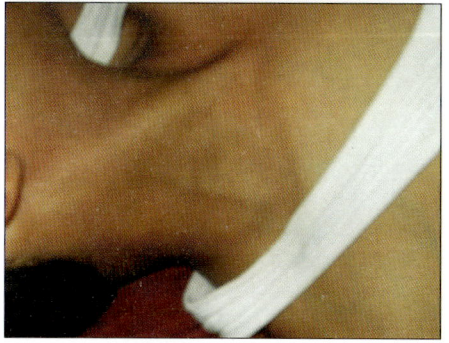

Hepatojugular reflex

Apex Heart Beat

1. Patient should be examined in the supine, sitting, and left lateral decubitus position.
2. Normal apical impulse occurs during early systole with an outward motion imparted to the chest wall.
3. Normal apex beat is palpable as brief outward impulse.

(Intersection of left mid-clavicular line and 5th intercostal space by the fingers.)

1. If the apex beat shifts more than 2 cm, it indicates left ventricular enlargement.
2. Double apical impulse caused by left ventricular hypertrophy and forceful left atrial contraction.

Examination of Chest Shape and Dimensions

Procedure: Measure the anteroposterior and lateral diameter of the chest wall.

Usually the ratio is 1:2.

POSTURE ANALYSIS OF THE PATIENT

Ask the patient to sit and stand.

Identify the patient's preferred sitting or standing posture.

A patient who has difficulty in breathing as a result of the COPD (chronic obstructive pulmonary diseases) usually leans forward on hands or forearms to stabilize and elevate the shoulder girdle to assist in inspiration.

Identify the patient sleeping posture. A patient with cardiopulmonary disorder usually prefers a head up rather than a fully recumbent position.

Also check the shoulder level is symmetrical or not.

Check the vertebral curves for any deformities like kyphosis, scoliosis.

ANALYZE THE CHEST SHAPE

Barrel Chest

The circumference of the upper chest appears larger than the lower chest. The sternum appears prominent, and the AP diameter of the chest is greater than the normal. Many patients with COPD develop this type of chest deformity.

Funnel Chest

Also called as pectus excavatum, the lower part of the sternum is depressed and the lower ribs are flared out, patients with this deformity are diaphragmatic breathers, excessive abdominal protrusion and little upper chest movement occurs in breathing.

Pigeon Chest

Also called pectus carinatum, the sternum is prominent and protrudes anteriorly.

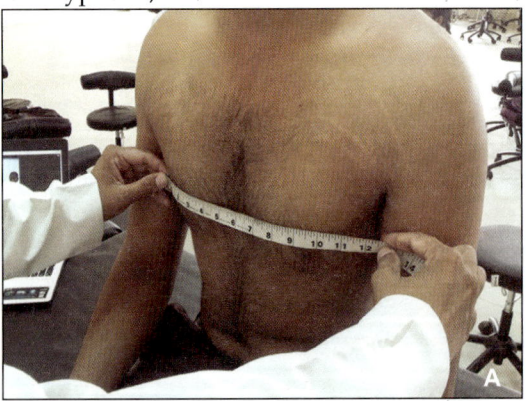 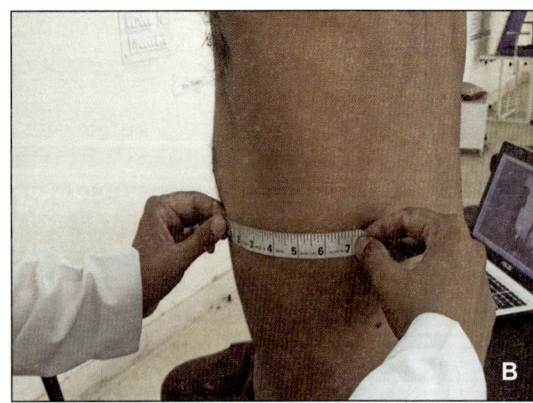

Technique of measuring (A) AP diameter of chest and (B) lateral diameter of chest

Examination of Breathing Pattern

Assess the rate, regularity and location of ventilation at rest and activity.

Normal respiratory rate in healthy adult is 16–20 cycles/min.

Check the inspiration and expiration ratio to identify the rhythm.

Usually, the ratio is 1:2 at rest and becomes 1:1 in activity.

A patient with COPD the ratio changes to 1:4 at rest.

The normal sequence of inspiration is:

1. The diaphragm contracts and descends and the abdomen rises.
2. This is followed by the lateral costal expansion as the ribs move up and out.
3. Finally, the upper chest rises.

Identify any difference in this pattern and report.

INTERPRETATION

The following terms are used to describe the abnormalities in the breathing pattern.

1. Dyspnea: Difficulty in breathing.

Grades of dyspnea

Grade	Description
1	Difficulty in breathing on unaccustomed activities
2	Difficulty in breathing on accustomed activities
3	Difficulty in breathing on ADL
4	Difficulty in breathing at rest
5	Difficulty in breathing on lying flat (orthopnea)

2. Tachypnea: Rapid, shallow breathing.
3. Bradypnea: Slow rate with shallow or normal depth and regular rhythm.
4. Hyperventilation: Deep, rapid respiration
5. Apnea: Cessation of breathing in the expiratory phase.

6. Apneusis: Cessation of breathing in inspiratory phase.
7. Cheyne-Stokes: Cycles of gradually increasing tidal volume and then a period of apnea.

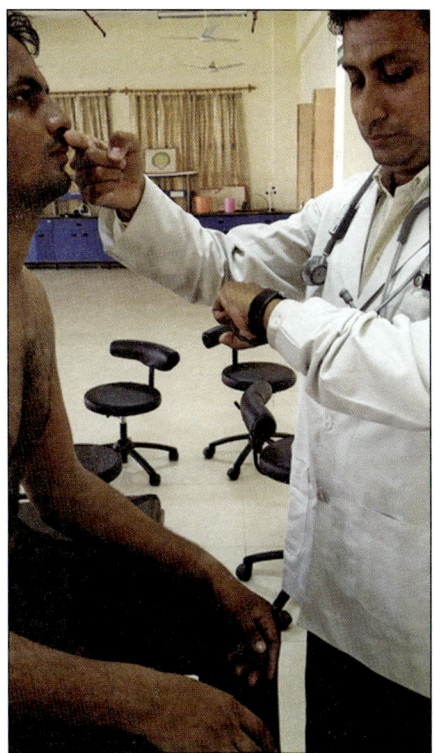

Examining the respiratory rate

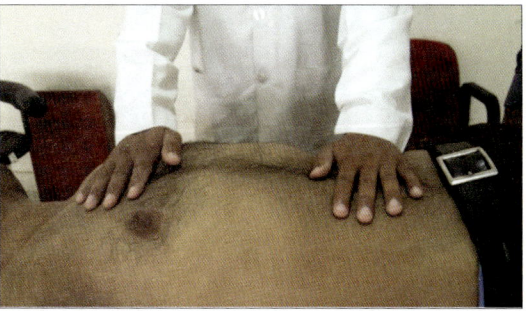

Examination of breathing pattern

Examination of Chest Mobility

Analysis of the symmetry of the moving chest is checked to identify the symmetrical mobility and expansion of the chest.

This gives information about the mobility of the chest and corresponds to areas to lung expansion.

Procedure: Explain the entire procedure to the patient.

Ask the patient to sit in front of you and relax.

Place your hands on the patient's chest and assess the excursion of each side of the thorax during inspiration and expiration.

Upper Lobe Expansion

To check the upper lobe expansion, face the patient.

Place the tips of your thumbs at the mid-sternal line at the sternal notch.

Extend your fingers above the clavicles.

Ask the patient fully exhale and then inhale deeply.

Middle Lobe Expansion

To check middle lobe expansion, continue to face the patient, place the tips of your thumbs at the xiphoid process and extend your fingers laterally around the ribs, again ask the patient to breathe deeply.

Lower Lobe Expansion

To check the lower lobe expansion, place the tips of your thumbs along the patient's back at the spinous processes and extend your fingers around the ribs. Ask the patient to breathe deeply.

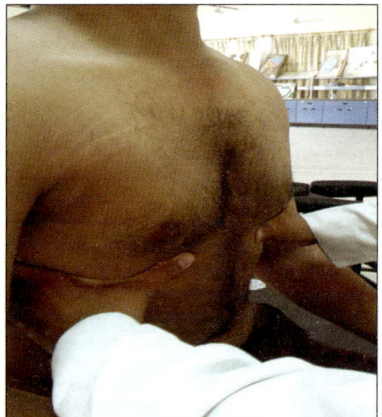

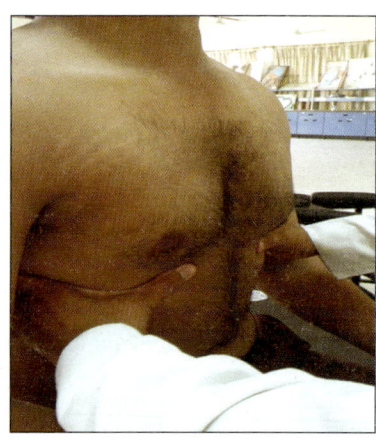

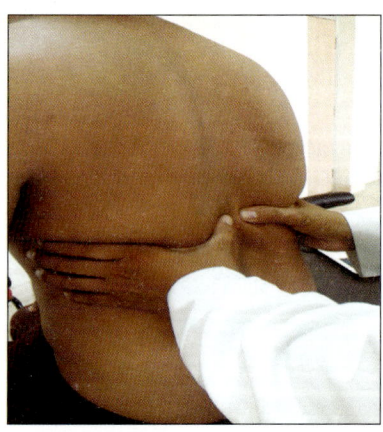

Percussion

This technique is used to assess lung density, the air-solid ratio in the lungs.

Procedure: Place the middle finger of the non-dominant hand flat against the chest wall along an intercostal space.

With the tip of middle finger of the opposite hand, firmly tap on the finger positioned on the chest wall.

Repeat the procedure on several points on the right and left and anterior and posterior aspects of the chest wall.

INFERENCE

This technique produces a resonance, the pitch varies with the density of the underlying tissue.

Report

Deter-minant	Right anterior	Right posterior	Left anterior	Left posterior
Result				

The sound is dull and flat, if there is greater than normal amount of solid matter as in the cases of tumor, consolidation in the lungs in comparison with the amount of air.

The sound is hyperresonant which is termed as tympanic, if there is a greater amount of air than the normal as in the case of emphysema.

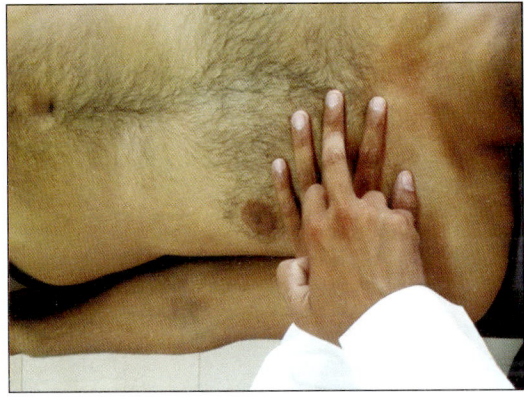

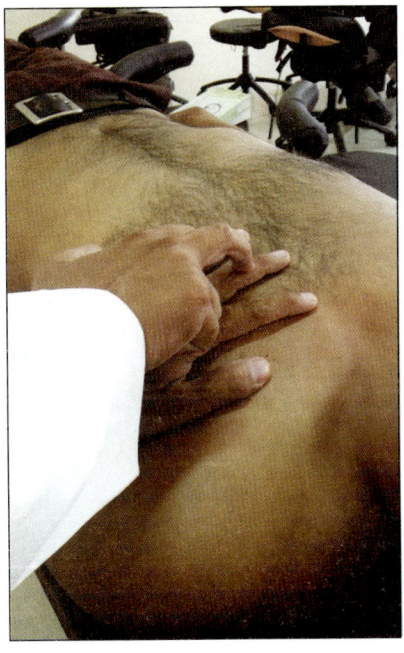

Auscultation Skills

AUSCULTATION OF BREATH SOUNDS

It is the technique of listening to sounds within the body, specifically to breath sounds during an examination of the lungs with the help of a sthethoscope which magnifies the sound.

Breath sounds occur because of movement of air in the airways during inspiration and expiration.

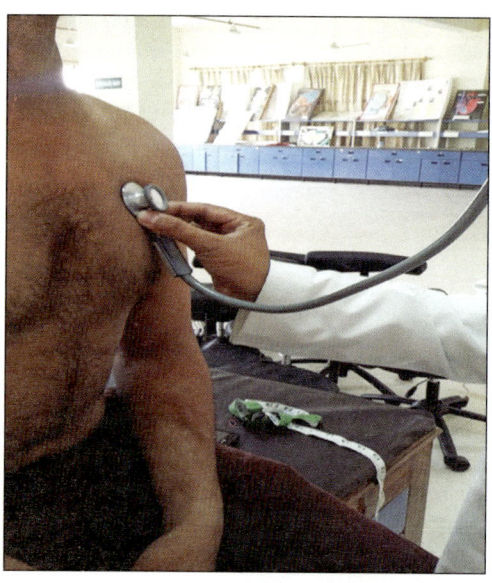
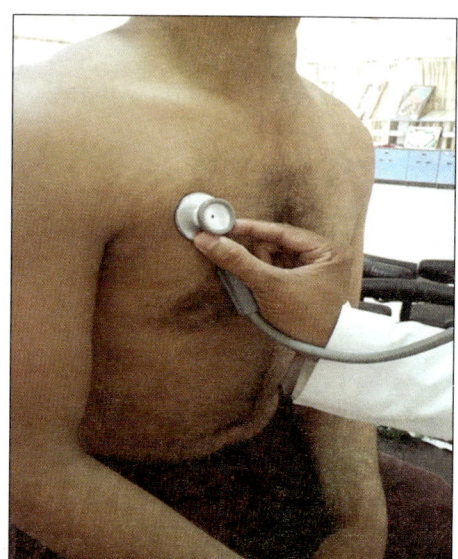
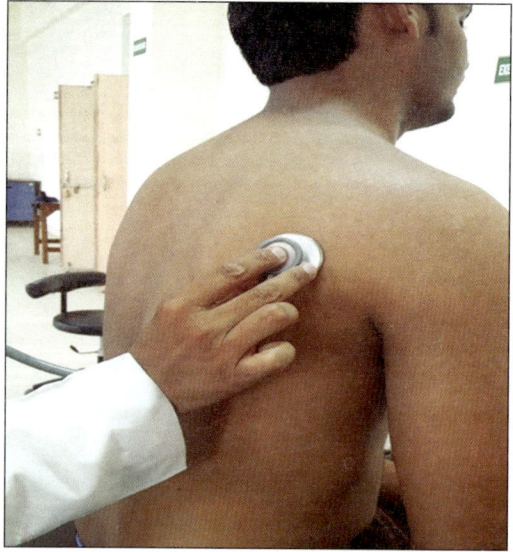
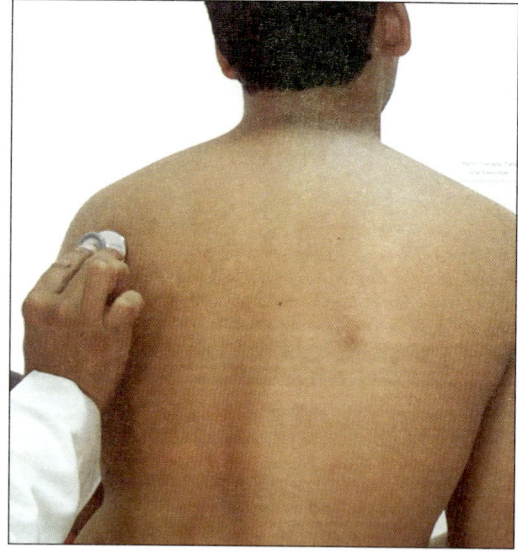

Breath sounds	Description	Result
Vesicular	Soft, low-pitched, breezy sounds heard over the most of the chest except at the trachea and between the scapulae, they are audible longer on inspiration	
Bronchial	Loud, hollow or tubular high-pitched sounds heard over the main stem bronchi and trachea. They are heard equally on inspiration and expiration, a slight pause is present between inspiration and expiration	
Broncho-vesicular	Softer than bronchial breath sounds equally heard on inspiration and expiration, but there is no pause. The sounds are heard in the supraclavicular, suprascapular and parasternal anteriorly and between the scapulae posteriorly	
Tracheal	Heard on trachea	

Procedure: When assessing the breath sounds, be sure the setting is quiet.

Have the patient assume a comfortable position to allow the access the chest wall.

Place the diaphragm of the stethoscope directly against the patient's skin along the anterior or posterior chest wall.

Make sure that the tube does not rub together or come in contact with clothing during auscultation.

For a systematic pattern, the stethoscope is placed on specific thoracic landmarks (T_2, T_6, T_{10}) along the right and left sides of the chest wall. Ask the patient to breathe in deeply and out quickly through the mouth.

AUSCULTATION OF HEART SOUNDS

Areas to Auscultate

1. Apex (mitral area) murmur originated from the MV are best heard.
2. Lower sternal edge (tricuspid area).
3. Lower left parasternal (4th intercostal space) murmur of AR is best heard.
4. Upper left parasternal (pulmonary area, 2nd left intercostal space).
5. Upper right parasternal (aortic area, 2nd right intercostal space murmurs arising from aortic valve area best heard).
6. Below the left clavile: Continuous murmur of PDA is best heard.
7. Posterior chest for bruits caused by bronchial collaterals in case of coarctation of the aorta.

Other areas: Abdominal aorta, renal arteries, carotid, femoral artery.

Examination of Cough

The strength, depth and length and frequency of the cough must be assessed:

- An effective cough is sharp and deep.
- A cough may be weak in pain or paralysis.
- A cough can be productive or non-productive.

If productive, then examine the sputum:

1. *Color:* Clear, yellow, green, blood-stained.
2. *Consistency:* Viscous, thin, frothy.
3. *Amount:* Minimal, copious.
4. *Odor:* No odor, foul smelling.

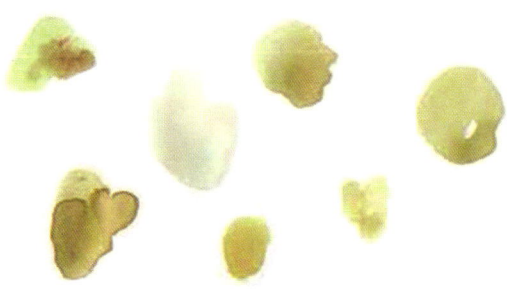

Target Heart Rate

Teaches you to monitor your heart rate.

Shows you how high your heart rate should be to get a good workout and increase cardiovascular fitness.

HELPS YOU BE AWARE TO NOT OVERWORK YOUR HEART

How do you find target heart rate?

FIRST, FIND YOUR RESTING HEART RATE

• Find your pulse, measure your heart beats for 10 seconds and multiply by 6 or measure for 15 seconds and multiply by 4.

• Your best resting heart rate is before you get out of bed in the morning.

MAXIMUM HEART RATE: 220–YOUR AGE

• This is the most your heart should ever beat.
• *Target heart rate:* (Maximum heart rate – Resting heart rate)(.7. + Resting heart rate = Target heart rate)

Resting heart rate	220–your age:	60–70%
My resting heart rate is:	220–___ = ____	

Heart Rate Target (10 Second Count)

Age	55%	60%	70%	80%	85%
15	19	21	24	27	29
20	18	20	23	27	28
25	18	19	23	26	28
30	17	19	22	25	27
35	17	19	22	25	26
40	17	18	21	24	26
45	16	18	20	23	25
50	16	17	20	23	24
55	15	17	19	22	23
60	15	16	19	21	23
65	14	16	18	21	22
70	14	15	18	20	21
75	13	15	17	19	21
80	13	14	16	19	20

24

Investigations

Examination of a Chest Radiograph

The chest X-ray can be of the following views:
1. Posteroanterior view (PA view)
2. Anteroposterior view (AP view)
3. Lateral view
4. Oblique or decubitus view

Precautions while Taking X-rays

When a physiotherapist visits X-ray department to observe the procedures, he/she must:

1. Stand behind the X-ray tube whenever possible.
2. Be as far away as possible from the X-ray tube.
3. Wear a lead rubber apron when necessary

READING A RADIOGRAPH

When reading a chest radiograph, it is important to follow some routine order so that no area is missed.

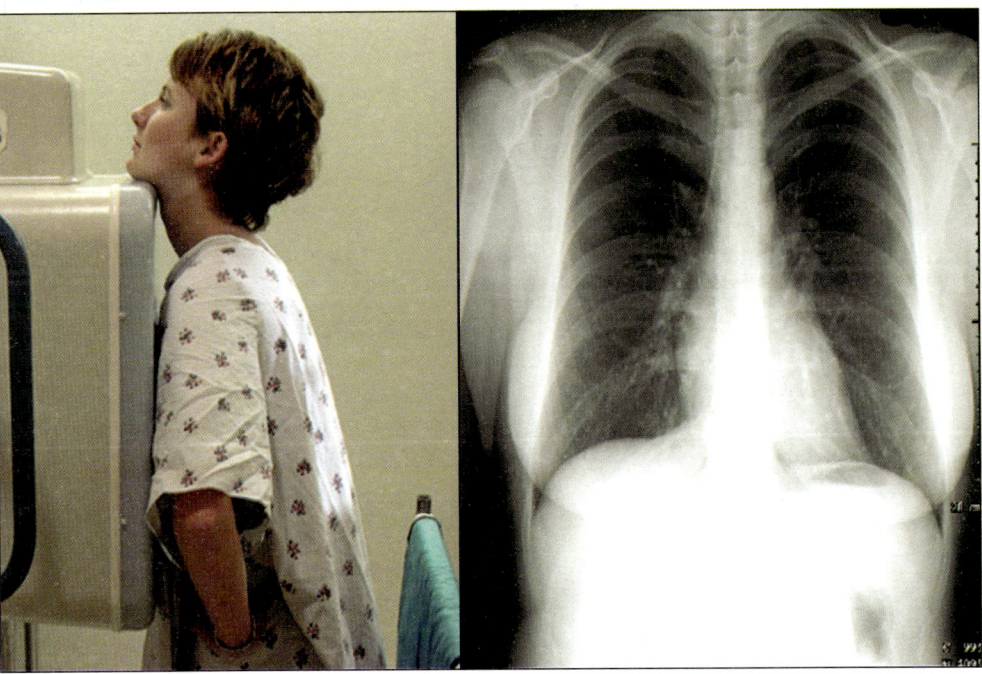

Posteroanterior view

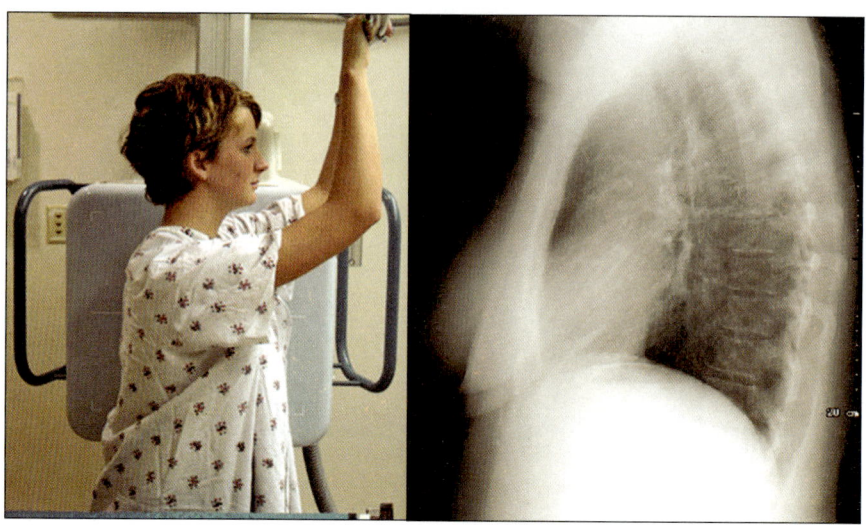

Lateral view

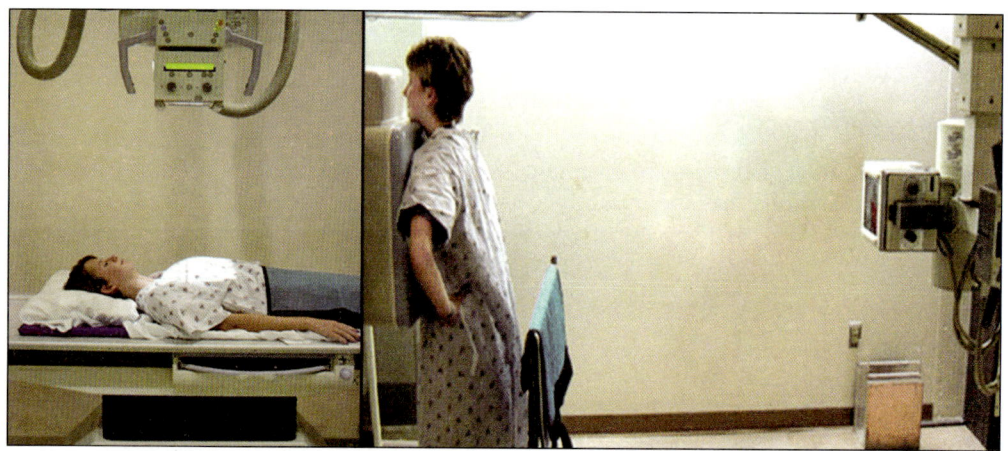

Anteroposterior view   Posteroanterior view

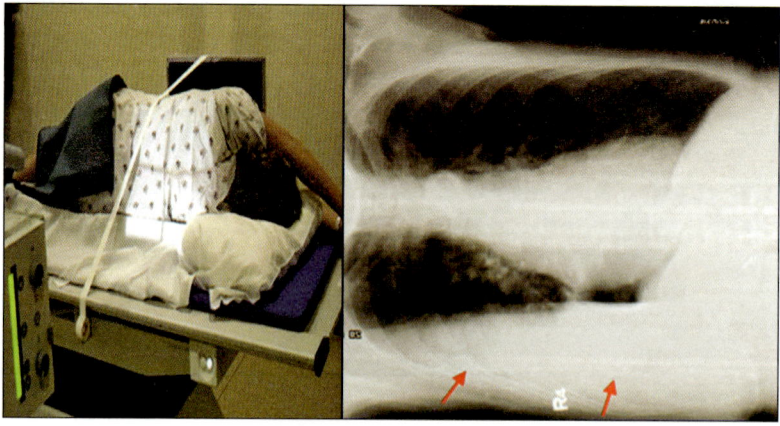

Decubitus/oblique view

Penetration

Adequate penetration of the patient by radiation is also required for a good film. On a good PA film, the thoracic spine disc spaces should be barely visible through the heart but bony details of the spine are not usually seen. On the other hand, penetration is sufficient that bronchovascular structures can usually be seen through the heart.

On the lateral view, you can look for proper penetration and inspiration by observing that the spine appears to be darken as you move caudally. This is due to more air in lung in the lower lobes and less chest wall. The sternum should be seen edge on and posteriorly you should see two sets of ribs.

Rotation: The technologists are usually very careful to X-ray the patient flat against the cassette. If there is rotation of the patient, the mediastinum may look very unusual. One can access patient rotation by observing the clavicular head and determining whether they are equal distance from the spinous process of the thoracic vertebral bodies.

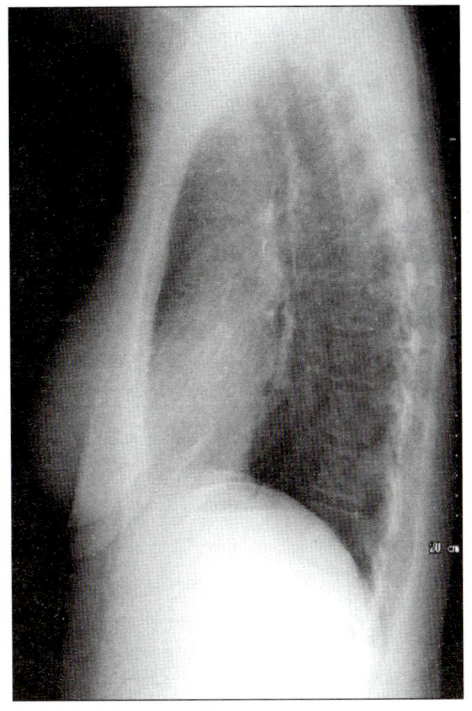

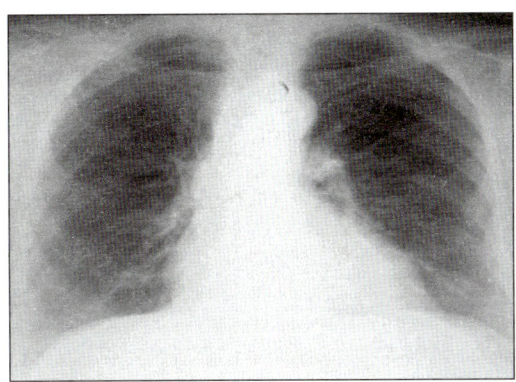

Underpenetrated X-ray

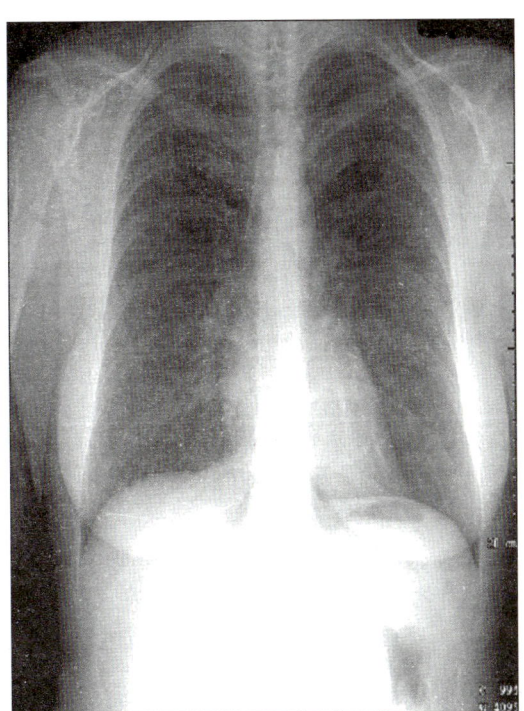

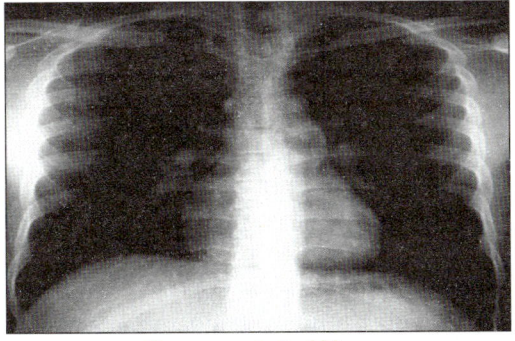

Over penetrated X-ray

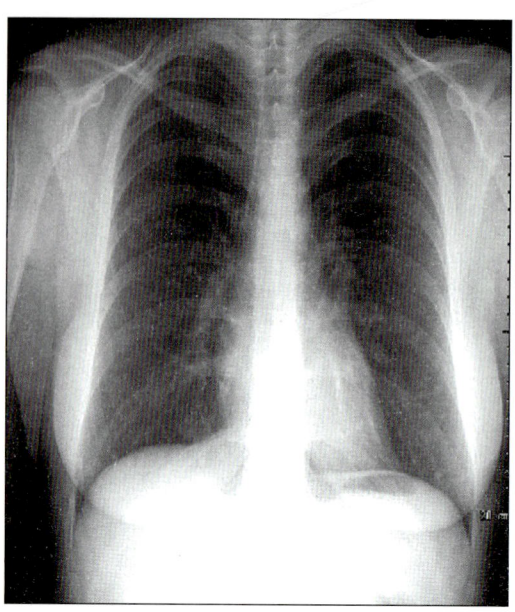

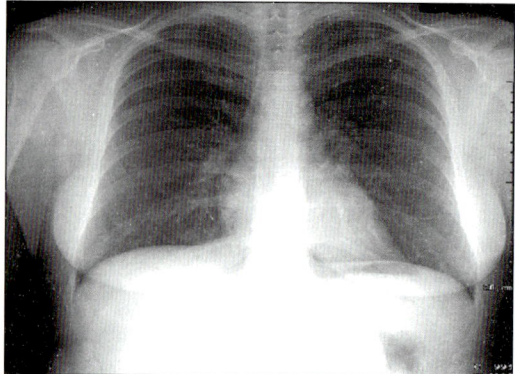

Inspiration

Interpretation of Chest X-Ray

When reading a chest X-ray, it is important to follow some routine order so that no area is missed.

1. Turn off stray lights, optimize room lighting, view images in order.
2. Patient data (name history #, age, sex, old films).
3. *Routine technique*: AP/PA, exposure, rotation, supine or erect.
4. *Trachea*: Midline or deviated, caliber, mass.
5. *Lungs*: Abnormal shadowing or lucency.
6. *Pulmonary vessels*: Artery or vein enlargement.
7. *Hila*: Masses, lymphadenopathy.
8. *Heart*: Thorax: heart width >2:1 ? Cardiac configuration?
9. Mediastinal contour—width? mass?
10. *Pleura*: Effusion, thickening, calcification.
11. *Bones*: Lesions or fractures.
12. *Soft tissues*: Don't miss a mastectomy.
13. *ICU films*: Identify tubes first and look for pneumothorax.

Inspiration

The patient should be examined in full inspiration. This greatly helps the radiologist to determine, if there are intrapulmonary abnormalities. The diaphragm should be found at about the level of the 8th–10th posterior rib or 5th–6th anterior rib on good inspiration.

Opacity

The basic diagnostic instance is to detect an abnormality. In both of the cases above, there is an abnormal opacity. It is most useful to state the diagnostic findings as specifically as possible, then try to put these together and construct a useful differential diagnosis using the clinical information to order it.

In each of the cases above, there is an abnormal opacity in the left upper lobe. In the case on the left, the opacity would best be described as a mass because it is well-defined. The case on the right has an opacity that is poorly defined. This is air space disease such as pneumonia.

Lobes and Fissures

On the PA chest X-ray, the minor fissure divides the right middle lobe from the right upper lobe and is sometimes not well seen. There is no minor fissure on the left. The major fissures are usually not well seen on the PA view because you are looking through them obliquely. If there is fluid in the fissure, it is occasionally manifested as a density at the lower lateral margin.

Mediastinum and Lungs

The physiotherapist needs to know both the structures within the mediastinum forming

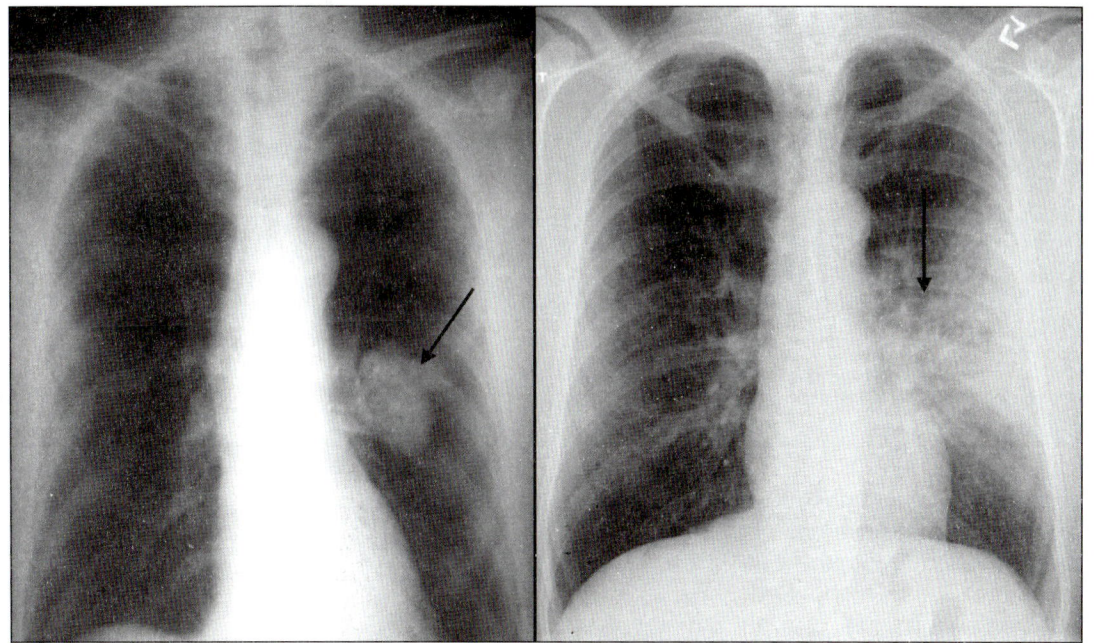

Opacity

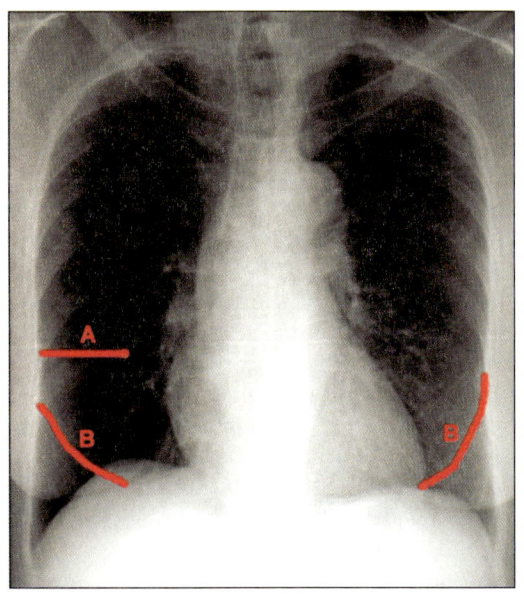

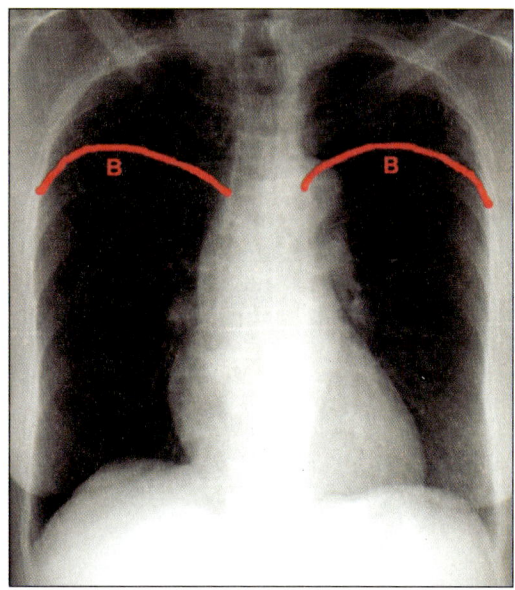

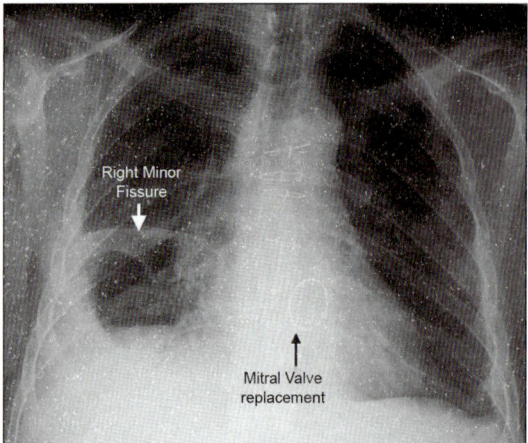

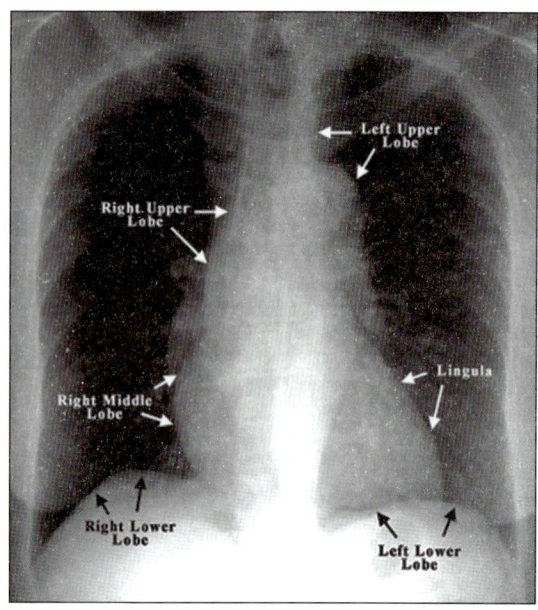

the mediastinal margins and the lobes of the lungs forming the margins of the lungs along the mediastinum and chest wall. If a mass or pneumonia "silhouettes" (obscures) a part of the lung/mediastinal margin, the therapist should be able to identify what part of the lung and what organ within the mediastinum are involved. The margins of the mediastinum are made up of the structures shown below. Trace the margin of the mediastinum with your eye all the way around the margin. Think of the mediastinal structures that comprise this interface. If the margin were abnormal you could diagnose the cause.

HEART SHADOW

Cardiothoracic Ratio

The simplest method of assessing the heart size is the ratio between the maximum diameter

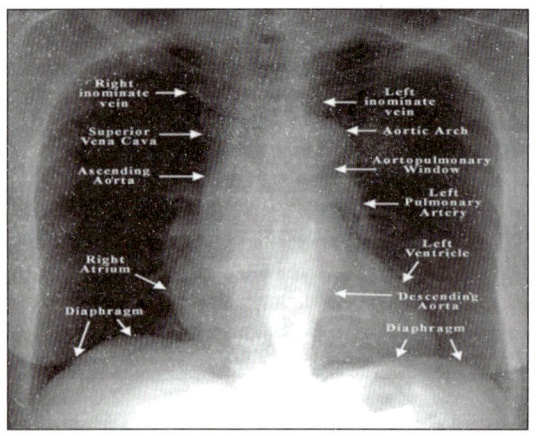

of the heart and the internal diameter of the rib cage. This is the cardiothoracic ratio and is normally 1: 2.

In an adult, a cardiac diameter grater than 15.5 cm is always considered abnormal.

Silhouette Sign

One of the most useful signs in chest radiology is the silhouette sign. This was described by Dr. Ben Felson. The silhouette sign is in essence elimination of the silhouette or loss of lung/soft tissue interface caused by a mass or fluid in the normally air-filled lung. In other words, if an intrathoracic opacity is in anatomic contact with, for example, the heart border, then the opacity will obscure that border. The sign is commonly applied to the heart, aorta, chest wall, and diaphragm. The location of this abnormality can help to determine the location anatomically.

Take a moment to review the makeup of the mediastinal margins and the lobes of the lungs that interface with the mediastinum. For the heart, the silhouette sign can be caused by an opacity in the RML (right middle lobe), lingula, anterior segment of the upper lobe, lower aspect of the oblique fissure, anterior mediastinum, and anterior portion of the pleural cavity. This contrasts with an opacity in the

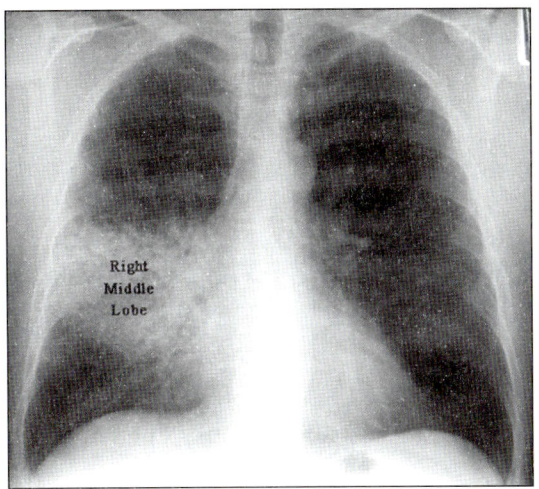

posterior pleural cavity, posterior mediastinum of lower lobes which cause an overlap and not an obliteration of the heart border. Therefore, both the presence and absence of this sign is useful in the localization of pathology.

AIR BRONCHOGRAM

An air bronchogram is a tubular outline of an airway made visible by filling of the surrounding alveoli by fluid or inflammatory exudates. Six causes of air bronchograms are: Lung consolidation, pulmonary edema, nonobstructive pulmonary atelectasis, severe interstitial disease, neoplasm, and normal expiration.

CONGESTIVE CARDIAC FAILURE

Congestive heart failure (CHF) is one of the most common abnormalities evaluated by chest X-ray. CHF occurs when the heart fails to maintain adequate forward flow. CHF may progress to pulmonary venous hypertension and pulmonary edema with leakage of fluid into the interstitium, alveoli and pleural space.

The earliest CXR finding of CHF is cardiomegaly, detected as an increased cardiothoracic

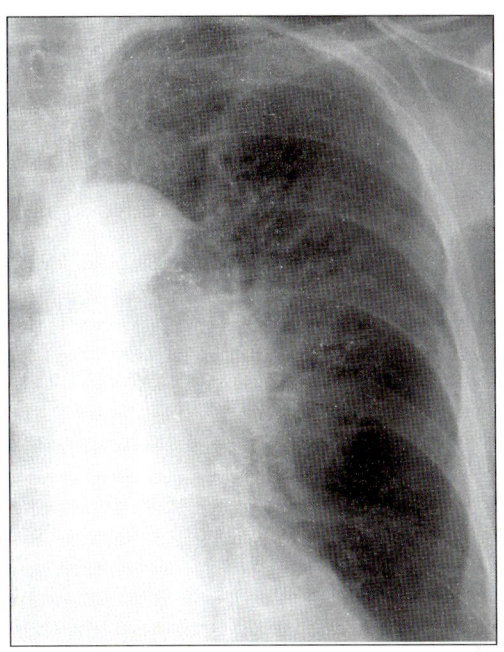

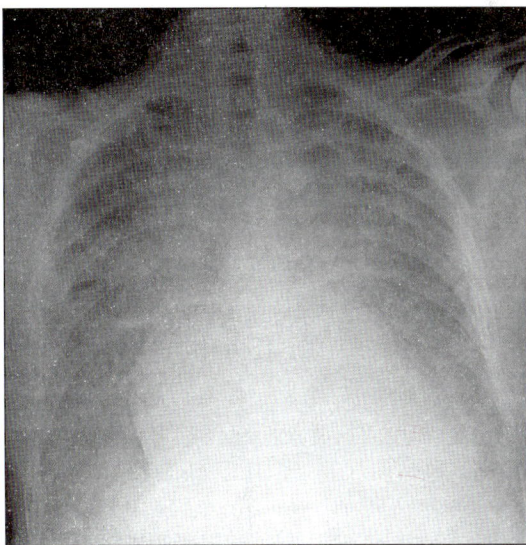

ratio (>50%). CXR is important in evaluating patients with CHF for development of pulmonary edema and evaluating response to therapy as well.

Basics of Electrocardiogram (ECG)

Definition: It is the graphical recording of the electrical potentials in the heart during cardiac cycle.
- These potentials are picked from the body surface, amplified and recorded by electrocardiograph.

Background: The conduction system of heart has four junctional tissues:
- Sinoatrial node
- Atrioventricular node
- Bundle of His and bundle branches
- Purkinje branches

CARDIAC CYCLE

The series of events occurring in the heart during each heart beat is called cardiac cycle. The various major series of events are:
- Contraction and relaxation of different chambers.
- Opening and closing of different valves.
- Occurrence of heart sounds.
- Blood flow through different chambers.

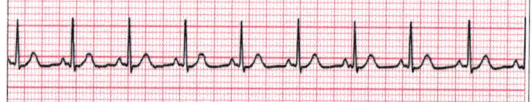

Events
- Atrial systole—0.1 sec
- Atrial diastole—0.7 sec
- Ventricular systole—0.3 sec
- Ventricular diastole—0.5 sec

Nodal Delay and Significance
- When the impulse reaches AV node, it is not immediately spreads into the bundle of His, but delays for 0.08 sec, this is called as 'nodal delay'.
- Nodal delay ensures that atrial contraction is completed before the ventricles begin contraction.
- This ensures proper filling of the ventricles.

What is an Electrical Event?

When the cardiac muscle has to contract, it must be excited, by depolarization, and when the muscle has to relax, it undergoes repolarization.

Thus in terms of electrical events, cardiac cycle includes:

- Atrial depolarization
- Atrial repolarization
- Ventricular depolarization
- Ventricular repolarization.

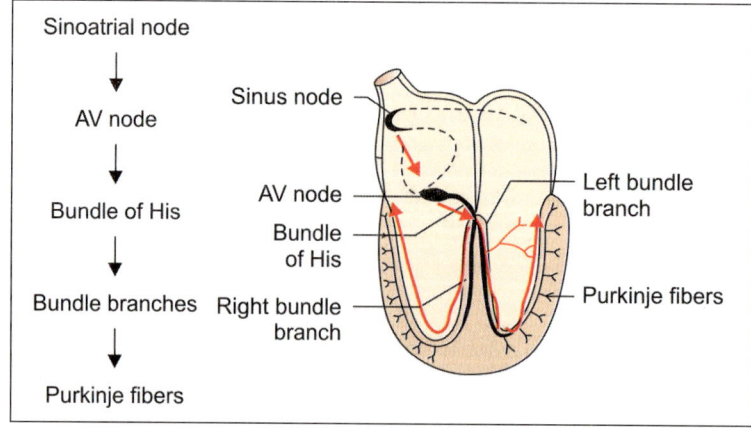

Normal impulse conduction

Components of ECG

- *Electrodes* "elecrodes are applied to right wrist, left wrist, left ankle.
  - ✎ Fourth electrode is applied to right ankle and is used for earthening purpose.
- *Lead selector:* By rotating the lead selector desired, lead can be obtained.
- *Amplifier:* It is used for the amplification of the electrical potentials.
- *Galvanometer:* Used for measuring the electrical potentials.
- *Thermal writing stylus:* It is attached to coil and it moves with the coil of galvanometer, this stylus is heated in the machine.

ECG Paper

It is a black paper coated with grey wax.

When heated stylus comes in contact with the wax, it melts and black graph is obtained.

- ECG paper has thick and thin lines horizontally and vertically.
- Thin lines are 1 mm apart and thick lines are 5 mm apart.
- Horizontally time is indicated. Vertically voltage is indicated.
- As the speed of ECG machine is 25 mm/sec,

1 mm=0.04 sec, 5 mm = 0.2 sec which denotes the duration.

Vertically voltage is indicated 10 mm = 1 mV

Lead

Lead is a closed circuit formed by connecting two points on the body surface and two terminals of ECG machine. Leads are of 2 types—unipolar and bipolar.

Unipolar Leads

In unipolar leads one electrode is exploring the electrical potentials and the other is indifferent electrode which remains neutral or at zero potential.

Unipolar leads are 2 types—unipolar limb leads and unipolar chest leads.

Placement of Electrodes for Unipolar Limb Leads

Lead	Exploring electrode connected to positive terminal of the machine	Indifferent electrodes to negative terminal of the machine
aVR	Rt. wrist	Left wrist and left foot
aVL	Left wrist	Right wrist and left foot
aVF	Left foot	Right and left wrist

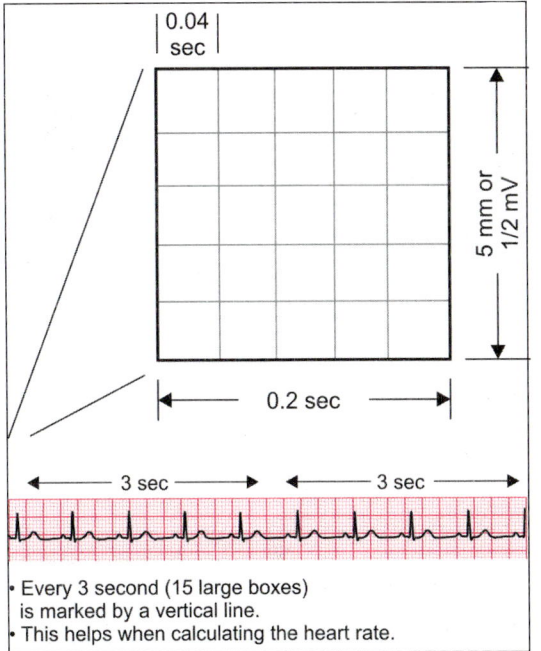

- Every 3 second (15 large boxes) is marked by a vertical line.
- This helps when calculating the heart rate.

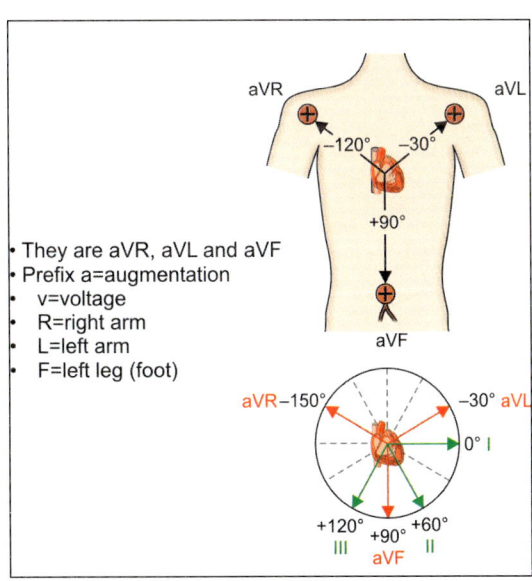

- They are aVR, aVL and aVF
- Prefix a=augmentation
  - v=voltage
  - R=right arm
  - L=left arm
  - F=left leg (foot)

Unipolar limb leads

Placement of Unipolar Chest Leads

- V1—4th inercostal space on the right border of sternum
- V2—4th intercostal space on the left border of sternum
- V3—between V2 and V4
- V5—5th intercostal space on the left anterior axillary line
- V6—5th intercostal space on the left mid axillary line

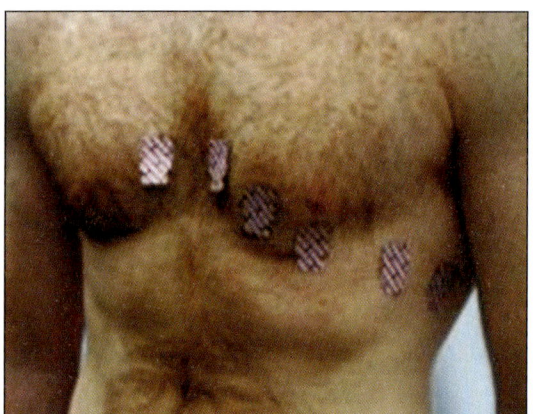

Placement of unipolar chest leads

Bipolar Limb Leads Placement

Lead	+ terminal	– terminal
I	LA	RA
II	LL	RA
III	LL	LA

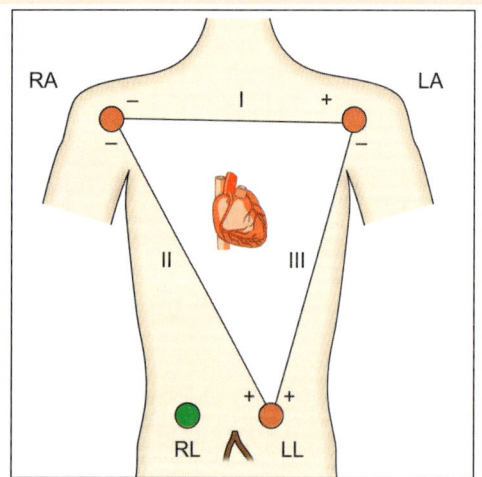

LA–left arm electrode, RA–right arm electrode, LL–left limb electrode

Eithoven's Triangle

- Eithoven's triangle is an imaginary equilateral triangle, the apices of which are formed by the roots of RA, LA, LL.
- Eithoven assumed that heart lies in the center of the triangle and produces the electric current which spreads to surface.
- Eithoven's law: Sum of potentials in leads I and III is equal to potentials produced in lead II.
- If potentials developed in any two leads are known, potential in third could be found.

> Therefore I +III =II

What do the Lead Inform?

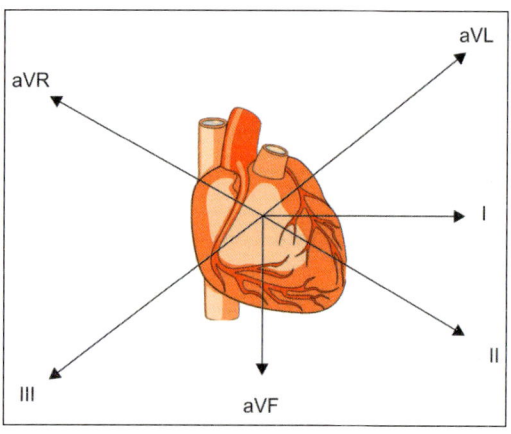

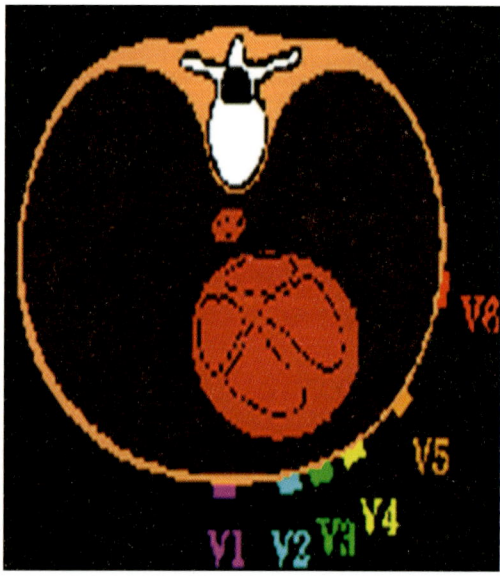

Chest Leads

V1 and V2 =look at the right ventricle

V3 and V4 =look at the septum between ventricles

V5 and V6 look at the anterior wall and lateral wall of left Ventricle

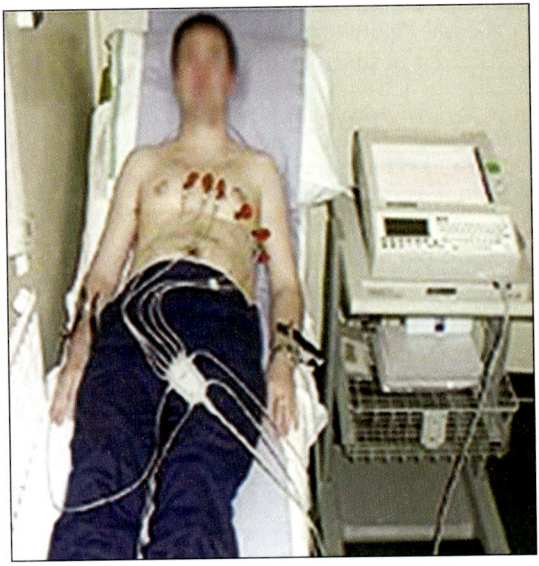

Recording an ECG

Recording an ECG

1. Explain procedure to the patient.
2. Check cables are connected.
3. Ensure surface is clean and dry.
4. Ensure electrodes are in good contact with the skin.
5. Enter patient data
6. Wait until the tracing is free from artifact.
7. Request the patient to lie still.
8. 'Push' button to start tracing.

Before disconnecting the leads, ensure the recording is:
- Free from artifact.
- Paper speed is 25 mm/sec.
- Normal standardization of 1 mV = 10 mm.
- Lead placement is correct.
- ECG is labelled correctly.

Why do a 12-Lead ECG?

- Monitor patients heart rate and rhythm.
- Evaluate the effects of disease or injury on heart function.
- Detect presence of ischemia/damage.
- Evaluate response to medications, e.g. anti-dysrhythmics.
- Obtain baseline recordings before, during and after surgical procedures.

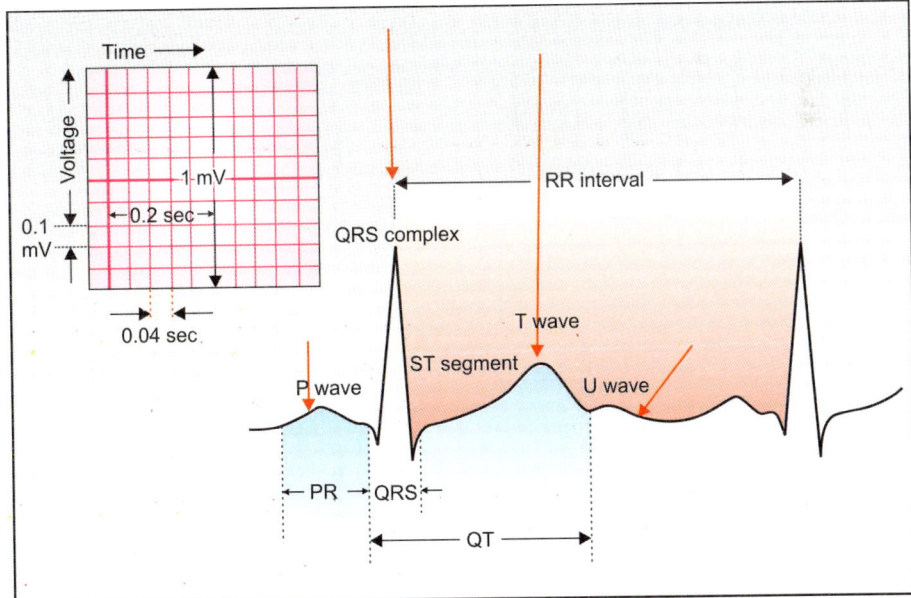

Normal ECG

Normal ECG

1. Normal electrocardiogram consists of P wave.
2. A 'QRS' complex.
3. A 'T' wave.
4. Sometimes U wave.

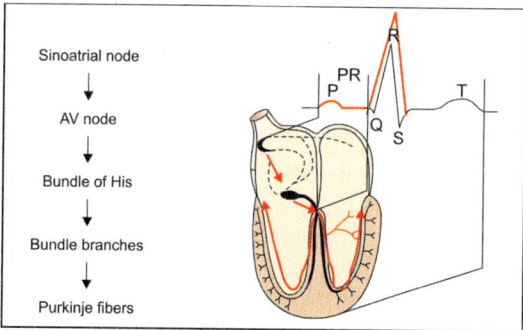

Impulse conduction and the ECG

P Wave

- P wave is produced by atrial depolarization.
- It is upright in leads I and II and is variable in lead III.
- Duration is less than 0.1 sec and amplitude is 0.25 mV.
- Shape is rounded.
- Normal P wave preceding a QRS complex with normal PR interval indicates that the heart is running in sinus rhythm.

P Wave Variables

- Tall and peaked P wave is called "P-pulmonale" seen in tricuspid valve stenosis.
- Broad and notched P wave is called as "P-mitrale", seen in mitral valve stenosis.
- Absent P wave indicates pacemaker is other than SAN.

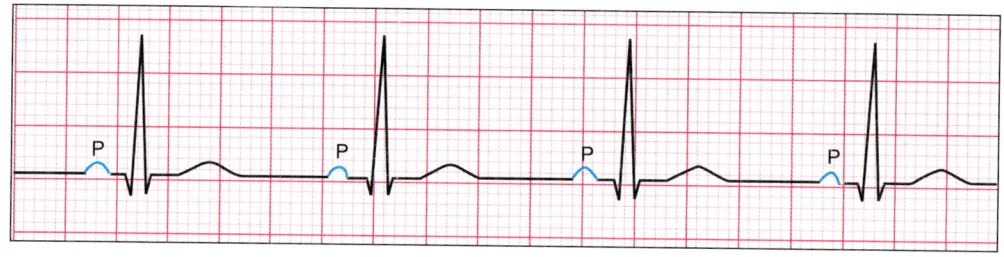

Normal P wave

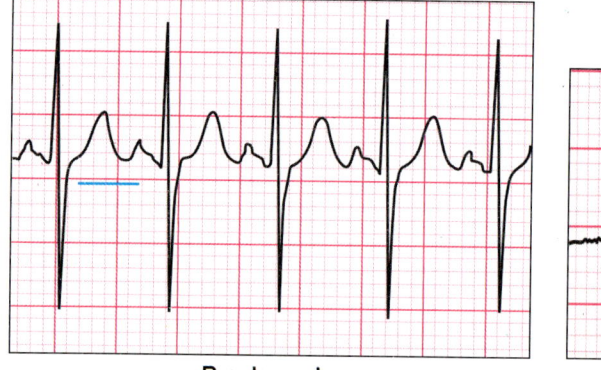

P-pulmonale

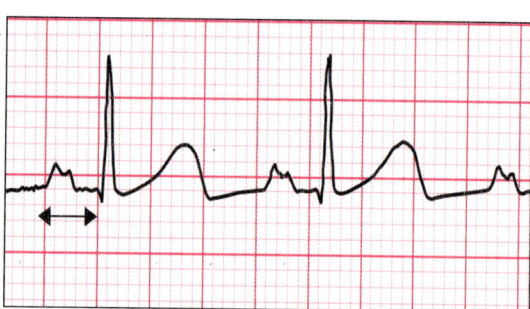

P-mitrale

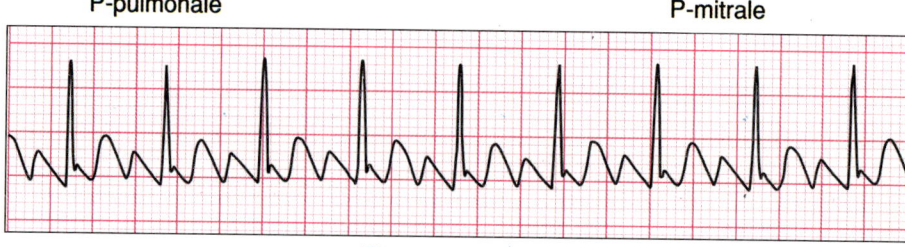

Flutter waves

- In atrial fibrillation, P wave is replaced by saw-tooth-shaped 'F' waves called flutter waves.

PR INTERVAL

- PR interval is also called as PQ interval.
- It is the interval between beginning of 'P' wave to beginning of QRS complex.
- Normal range is 0.12 to 0.2 sec and average 0.16 sec.

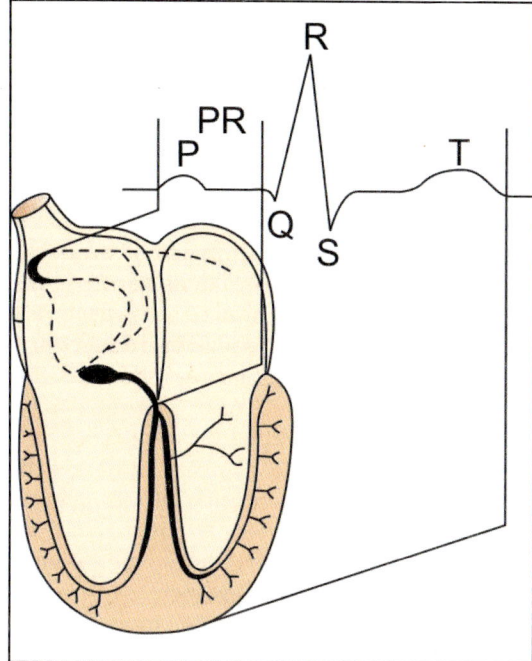

- Atrial depolarization + delay in AV junction (AV node/bundle of His) (delay allows time for the atria to contract before the ventricles contract)
- Rise in PR interval occurs in heart block.

QRS COMPLEX

It is the sequence of deflections due to ventricular depolarization.
  Nomenclature:
- Q=first '-'ve deflection of QRS complex
- R=first '+'ve deflection of QRS complex
- S='-'ve deflection,
  Duration: It is from beginning of Q wave to end of S wave. It is 0.08 to 0.1 sec [2–2.5 mm]

Shape of QRS Complex

Limb Leads

The ECG machine is arranged so that when a depolarization wave spreads towards a lead, the stylus moves upwards, and when it spreads away from the lead the stylus moves downwards.

- If the QRS complex is predominantly upward or positive (i.e. the R wave is greater than S wave), the depolarization is moving towards that lead.
- If predominantly downward or negative (S wave greater than R wave), the depolarization is moving away from that lead.
- When the depolarization wave is moving at right angles to the lead, the R and S waves are of equal size.

Cardiac Axis

- Normal cardiac axis is downward and to the left, i.e. the wave of depolarization travels from the right atrium towards the left ventricle.
- When an electrical impulse travels towards a positive electrode, there will be a positive deflection on the ECG.
- If the impulse travels away from the positive electrode, a negative deflection will be seen.
- Leads aVR and II look at the heart from opposite directions.
- Seen from the front, the depolarization wave normally spreads through the ventricles from 11'o clock to 5'o clock.

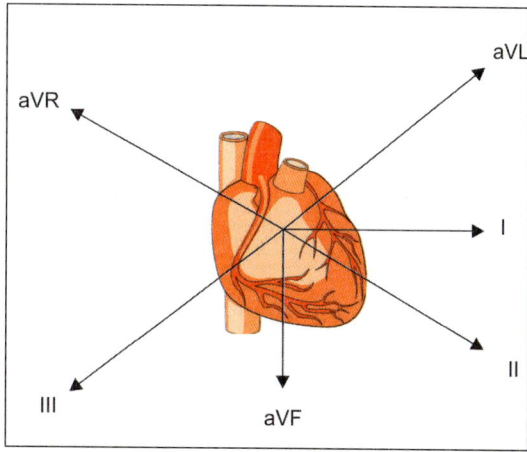

- So the deflections in lead aVR are normally mainly downward [negative] and in lead II mainly upward [positive].
- The average direction of spread of the depolarization wave through the ventricles as seen from the front is called the 'cardiac axis'.
- The direction of the axis can be derived most easily from QRS complexes in leads I, II, III.
- A normal 11'o clock to 5'o clock axis means that the depolarizing wave is spreading towards leads I, II, III and is, therefore, upward deflection in these leads, the deflection will be greater in lead II than I and III.
- If the right ventricle is hypertrophied, the axis will swing towards the right, the deflection in lead I becomes negative, and the deflection in lead III will become more positive [upward].
- This is called right axis deviation and is associated with pulmonary conditions and with congenital heart disorders.
- When the left ventricle is hypertrophied, the axis may swing to the left, so the QRS complex becomes predominantly negative in lead III. This is called as 'left axis deviation'.
- Left axis deviation is not significant until QRS deflection is also predominantly negative in lead II, and the problem is mainly conduction defect rather than left ventricle hypertrophy.

QRS Complex in Chest Leads

The shape of the QRS complex in the chest leads is determined by:
- The septum between the ventricles is depolarized before the walls of the ventricles, and the depolarization wave spreads across the septum from left to right.
- In the normal heart, there is more muscle in the wall of the left ventricle than that of right ventricle, hence left ventricle has more influence on ECG pattern than right ventricle.
- Leads V1 and V2 look at the right ventricle, leads V3 and V4 look at the septum, and leads V5 and V6 at the left ventricle.

Stage I

- In a right ventricular lead, the deflection is first upwards (R) as the septum is depolarized.
- In a left ventricular lead, the deflection is first downwards, there is a small Q wave called "septal Q wave".

Stage II

- In a right ventricular lead (V1 and V2), there is a downward deflection(s) as the main muscle is depolarized.
- In a left ventricular lead, there is an upward deflection (R) as the ventricular muscle is depolarized.
- When the whole of the myocardium is depolarized the ECG returns to baseline.
- The QRS complex in the chest leads shows a progression from lead V1, where it is predominantly downward, to lead V6, where it is predominantly upward.
- The "transition point", where the R and S waves are equal, indicates the position of the interventricular septum.
- If the right ventricle is enlarged and occupies more of the pericardium than normal, then the transition point will move from its normal position of leads V3–V4 to leads V4–V5 or V5–V6, seen from below, the heart can be thought of as having rotated in a clockwise direction, in ECG it is characteristic of chronic lung disease.

Variation of QRS Complex

- Abnormal wide QRS complex indicates the presence of bundle branch block or extra systoles.
- If the height of the QRS complex is abnormally high, then it indicates an increased muscle mass in either ventricle [hypertrophy].
- Q waves greater than one small square in width and at least 2 mm deep indicate myocardial infarction.

ST Segment

- This is the interval between the end of S wave and beginning of T wave.
- Normally, it is isoelectric, i.e. in the same line with the RQ segment.
- Depression by ½ mm or elevation by 1–2 mm is normal.

Variations of ST Segment

- Elevation of ST segment indicates acute myocardial injury, usually due to recent infarction or due to pericarditis.
- Horizontal depression of ST segment, associated with an upright T wave, is usually a sign of infarction.

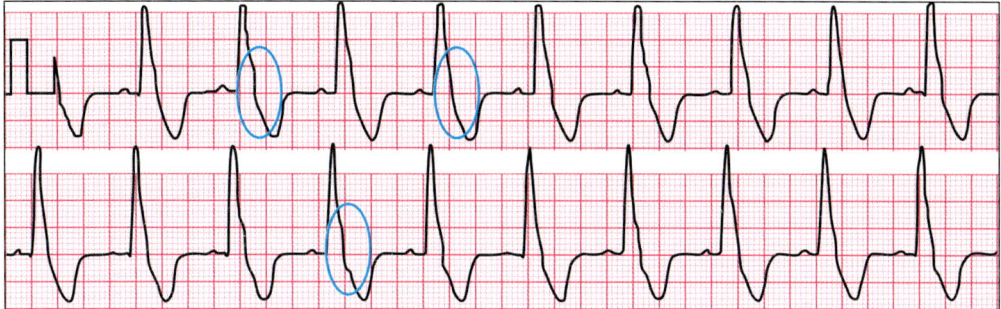

Variation of QRS complex

- When the ECG at rest is normal, ST depression can be seen during exercise, when effort induces angina.
- Downsloping, as opposed to horizontally depressed, ST segment are usually due to treatment with 'D' igoxin.

T WAVE

- It is the deflection following the QRS complex and is produced due to ventricular repolarisation.
- Should be in the same direction as and smaller than the QRS complex.
- Shape: A symmetrical gradual upstroke and steep downstroke.

Inverted T Wave

Inverted T wave is seen in following conditions:
- Normally seen in leads aVR and V1.
- Ischemia.
- Ventricular hypertrophy.
- Bundle branch block.
- Digoxin treatment.

QT Interval

- It is measured from beginning of Q wave to end of T wave.
- Normal QT interval is less than 0.42 sec.

Variations of QT Interval

Short QT interval is seen in electrolyte abnormalities.

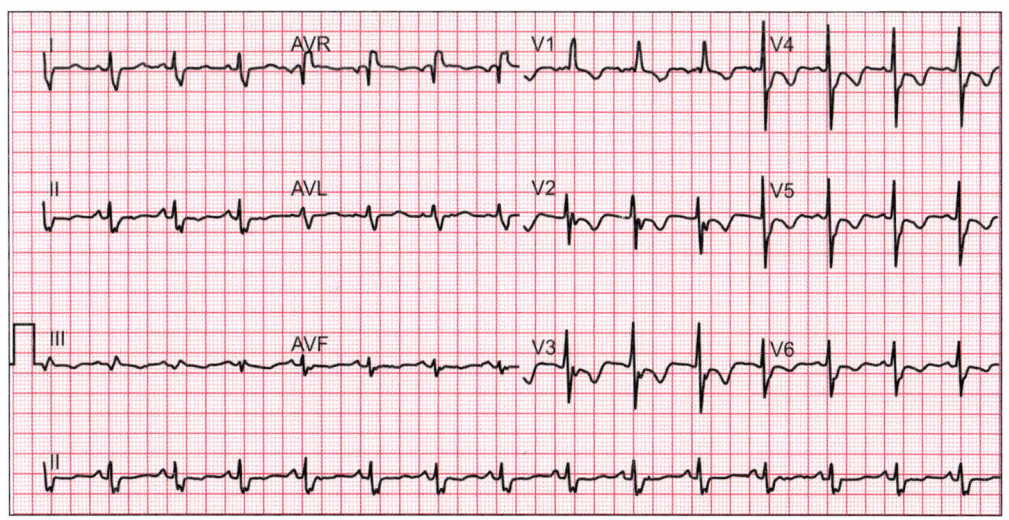

Inverted T wave

Counting of Heart Rate

Relationship between the number of large squares covered by RR interval and the heart rate can be found

RR interval [large squares]	Heart rate
1	300
2	150
3	100
4	75
5	60
6	50

Another method of counting heart rate is:
1. First count the small squares between two successive R waves.
2. Divide 1500 by the number of squares.

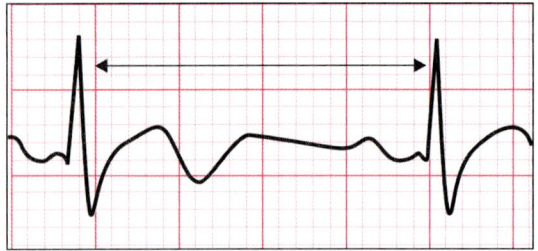

Inverted T wave

Electrodiagnosis SD Curve

Aim: To plot SD curve for various major nerves in the body.

Apparatus: Electrical stimulator with diagnostic interupted galvanic current facility.
1. Skin resistance tray consisting of:
   a. Bowl of tap water
   b. Soap
   c. Macintosh
   d. Kidney tray / plastic bowl
   e. Towels and tissue paper
2. Treatment tray consisting of:
   a. Leads
   b. Electrodes
   c. Lint
   d. 1% saline warm water in plastic bowl
   e. Supporting pads, pillows
   f. Cotton
   g. Talcum powder
   h. Vaseline
   i. Towels
   j. Velcrow straps/adhesive plaster

PROCEDURE

1. Greet the patient
2. Introduce yourself to the patient.
3. Take preliminary introduction and brief history from the patient.

METHOD OF APPLICATION

Preparation of the Apparatus

- First an electric stimulator with diagnostic interupted galvanic current facility is selected.
- Make sure that all the wires from mains to plug box and to the machine are intact and properly insulated.
- Check the leads for any breaks in the insulation.
- Test the machine by attaching leads and electrodes to the terminals and feel the current by switching 'on' the machine and increasing the intensity.
- Make sure that before 'on' or 'off' an apparatus, all the knobs of intensity are at 'zero'.
- Select the appropriate and suitable electrode.
- The electrodes should be properly linted.
- The inactive electrode is applied to some convenient area usually on the midline of the body, or over the origin of the muscle.
- The active electrode is usually a pen electrode.
- To assess a nerve, we choose a proximal muscle and a distal muscle supplied by that nerve in its course.
- The active pen electrode is placed over the motor point of the muscle to be tested.

- The longest pulse duration is choosen first and the intensity of the current is increased until the minimum observable contraction is obtained.
- Note the intensity of current and reduce the intensity to zero.
- Now shift the duration to second longest duration and repeat the procedure.
- Note the intensity of current required to get the similar and equal contraction for various durations as described below.

Duration (millisec)	Intensity (milliamp)
300	
100	
30	
10	
3	
1	
0.3	
0.1	
0.03	
0.01	

- Now plot on a graph paper by taking duration on X-axis and intensity in Y-axis.
- SD curve is drawn by connecting the plotted points.

Inference

- By plotting the curve, we can know whether a nerve is:
    a. Completely innervated
    b. Completely denervated
    c. Partially innervated and partially denervated
- Then, find the rheobase and chronaxie.
- *Rheobase*: The rheobase is the smallest current that will produce a muscle contraction.
- *Chronaxie*: It is the duration of the shortest impulse that will produce a response with a current of double rheobase.

Winding off

Remove the electrodes and clean the area with a tissue or cotton.

Check the area for any adverse effects, if found any, document it and report to the HOD or your supervisor.

Advantages

- Can determine the extent of degeneration in the nerve.
- To identify and estimate prognosis
- To plan the therapy.

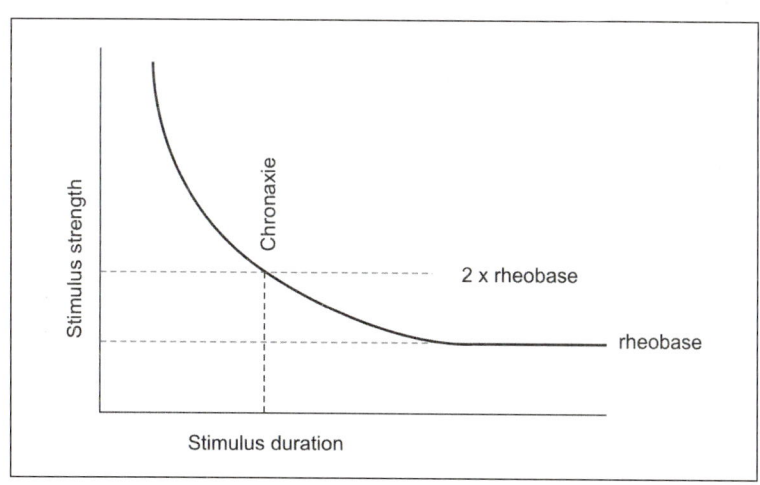

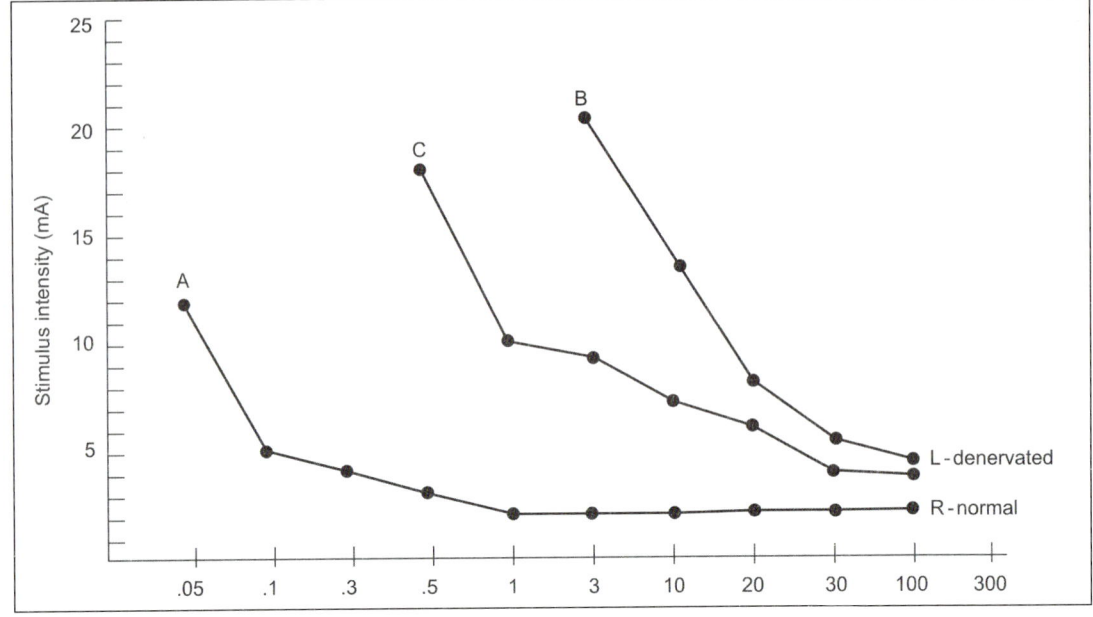

FG Test

Aim: To identify the amount, the regeneration/ or to find out whether the given muscles is innervated or denervated.

Apparatus

1. Electrical stimulator with diagnostic interrupted galvanic current and surged faradic current facility.
2. Skin resistance tray consisting of:

   a. Bowl of tap water
   b. Soap
   c. Macintosh
   d. Kidney tray/plastic bowl
   e. Towels and tissue paper

3. Treatment tray consisting of:

   a. Leads
   b. Pen and plate/carbon electordes
   c. Lint
   d. Conduction gel
   e. 1% saline warm water in plastic bowl.
   f. Supporting pads, pillows

   g. Cotton
   h. Talcum powder
   i. Vaseline
   j. Towels
   k. Velcrow straps/adhesive plaster.

Procedure

1. Greet the patient.
2. Introduce yourself to the patient.
3. Take preliminery introduction and brief history from the patient.
4. Assess the patient and judge which muscles to be stimulated.

Preparation of Apparatus

a. First, a low frequency electronic stimulator with surged faradic and interrupted galvanic current facility is selected.
b. Make sure that all the wires from the mains to plug box and to the machine are intact and properly insulated.

c. Check the leads for any breaks in the insulation

d. Test the machine by attaching leads and electordes to the terminals and feel the current by switching 'on' the machine and increasing the intensity.

e. Make sure that before starting 'on' or 'off' an apparatus, all intensity knobs are at zero.

f. Select the appropriate and suitable electrodes.

g. The electrodes should be properly linted or stuffed in sponge pad.

h. If using a carbon electrode, use good amount of conduction gel.

i. It should be noted that there should be at least eight layers of folds in lint covering the electrode.

j. The layers should be crease free and the lint pad should be 1 cm greater all around that of the electrodes.

k. The lint pads are soaked in 1% saline or tap water to devrease the resistance.

Preparation of Patient

a. Place the patient in supine lying or a suitable and comfortable position with a pillow under the head.

b. Explain briefly the entire procedure of the treatment.

c. Describe the patient the sensation he would feel during the treatment.

d. To make the patient feel confident, show the type of contraction by placing the electrodes first on your body.

e. Check the sensations of the skin to be treated.

f. The part to be treated must be exposed.

g. The skin resistance should be reduced by washing the area with soap and water.

h. Avoid placing the electrodes over or near the breaks or abrasions of skin. If it is inevitable and necessary, then the broken or abrased kin is protected by applying vaseline or petroleum jelly.

i. The indifferent electrode isplaced in position by applying strap or adhesive bandage.

Method of Application

In order to achieve the stimulation of motor points, two techniques are used

1. **Labile method:** The plate or carbon electrode connected to cathode is placed over the origin of the muscle and the muscle in turn is stimulated with a pen electrode connected to anode which is active.

   Note: Muscle contractions are often obtained mostly if the active electrode is connected to anode, but this is not the case always, each patient should be tested to determine whether anode or cathode is used for active electrode

2. **Stabile method:** Here two plates or carbon electrodes are used, one placed at origin of the muscle and the other at the insertion of the muscle to be stimulated. This technique is used for stimulating deep and large muscles.

Technique

Stimulate the muscle to be tested with the following parameters first by IG current and then by surged faradic current.

Interupted Galvanic Current

- Impulse—rectangular
- Duration—100 ms, but sometimes, the duration is increased to 300 ms depending upon the status of the muscle and differs with each patient.
- Intensity—sufficient for getting a good contraction.

Surged Faradic Current

Parameter	Description
Type	Surged faradism
Frequency	50–100 Hz
Pulse	Triangular
Duration	0.1–1 ms
On-off time	1:4
Amplitude (intensity)	Sufficient for muscle contraction

Inference

1. Note the intensity taken to get a minimal contraction for IG and surged faradic currents.
2. If IG current takes a lesser intensity to stimulate and the muscle does not respond to surged faradic, then the muscle is denervated.
3. If surged faradic current takes a lesser intensity than IG current to get a minimal contraction in the muscle, then the muscle is innervated.

Winding Off

Inspect the treatment area for any signs of adverse effects and if found any, document it.

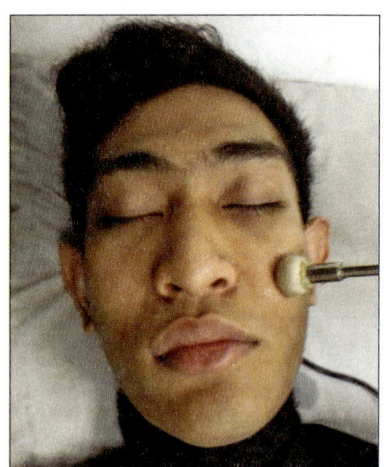

Nerve Conduction Velocity

- It is a rate of acceleration through which impulses travel down the neuronal pathway.
- It depends upon the fibre diameter and intermodal distance.
- The larger the axon, thicker the myelin sheath, longer the intermodal distance and faster the nerve conduction velocity.

CONDUCTION VELOCITY

It is a measurement made by the stimulating and recording electrodes from the two different sites along the course of nerve.

$$\text{Conduction velocity} = \frac{\text{Distance between two sites}}{\text{Distance in conduction times between two sides}}$$

Factors Affecting Nerve Conduction Velocity

- Age
- Sex
- Height
- Pathological delays occur with various medical conditions (carpal tunnel syndrome, nerve injuries, demyelinating neuropathies, etc.)
- Temperature
- The upper limb nerve conduction velocity is higher compared to lower limb nerve conduction velocity.

Principles of Motor Nerve Conduction

- It is performed by electrical stimulation of a peripheral nerve and recording from the muscle supplied by this nerve.
- For prevention of hyperpolarisation effect of anodal conduction block, supramaximal stimulation is done keeping cathode close to active recording electrode.
- The surface recording electrodes are placed in belly tendon keeping active electrode closer to motor point and reference to the tendon.
- The ground electrodes are kept between stimulating and recording electrodes.
- The healthy nerve requires surface stimulation of:
    - ✍ Square wave pulse—0.1 ms and intensity— 5–40 mA.

Formula of motor nerve conduction $= \dfrac{D}{PL - DL}$

Where   PL = Proximal latency.
          DL = Distal latency.
          D = Distance between proximal and distal stimulation in mm.

The measurement of motor nerve conduction includes:

a. *Onset latency:* The time it takes for the electrical impulse to travel from stimulation to the recording site is measured and this

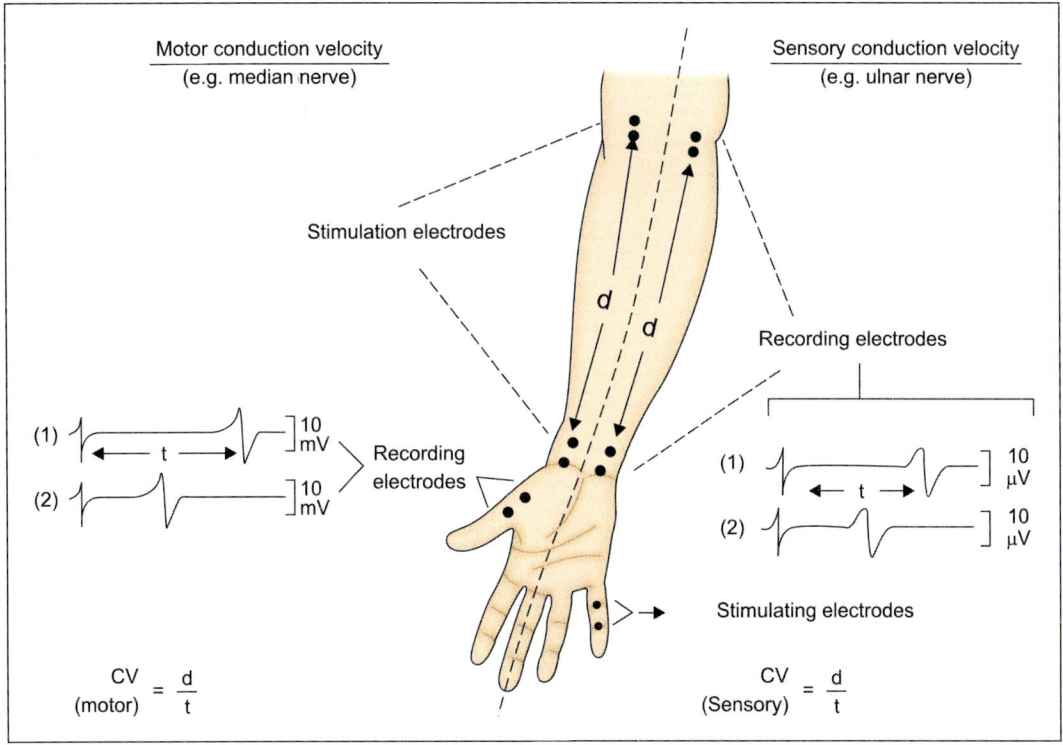

Motor conduction velocity
(e.g. median nerve)

Sensory conduction velocity
(e.g. ulnar nerve)

Stimulation electrodes

Recording electrodes

Recording electrodes

Stimulating electrodes

$$\underset{(motor)}{CV} = \frac{d}{t}$$

$$\underset{(Sensory)}{CV} = \frac{d}{t}$$

Diagram showing electrode placement with distance and time in motor conduction velocity (motor nerve) and sensory conduction velocity (ulnar nerve).

value is called the latency and is measured in milliseconds.

b. *Duration:* The time of response.

c. *Amplitude of compound muscle action potential:* The size of the response.

d. Nerve conduction velocity.

Principles of Sensory Nerve Conduction

- It is performed by electrical stimulation of a peripheral nerve and recording from the sensory portion of the nerve.
- The sensory receptors are innervated by different types of nerve fibres.
  - ↳ Proprioceptors: Type IA and IB, II sensory fibres.
  - ↳ Mechanoreceptors: Type II and III sensory fibres.
  - ↳ Nociceptors: Type III and type IV sensory fibres.

- It can be measured by 2 types:
  a. Orthodromically
  b. Antidromically
  ↳ In orthodromic conduction, distal nerve is stimulated and nerve action potential is recorded at the proximal nerve.
  ↳ In antidromically conduction, proximal nerve is stimulated and nerve action potential is recorded distally.
- The measurement of sensory nerve conduction includes:
  a. Onset latency
  b. Duration
  c. Amplitude of sensory nerve action potential.
  d. Nerve conduction velocity.

Procedure of Nerve Conduction Velocity

- It is used to determine the severity of nerve damage.

- Place the 2 electrodes on the nerve to be tested on the patient's skin surface.
- The one electrode is stimulated and other will record the impulse travel through the nerve.
- The distance between stimulating and receiving electrodes is divided by the impulse latency and conduction velocities.

Normal Values for Motor and Sensory Conduction of Various Nerves

Motor	Sensory
Ulnar and median nerves = 50–60 m/s	Ulnar and median nerves = 60–70 m/s
Common peroneal nerve = 45–55 m/s	Common peroneal nerve = 50–70 m/s

Electromyography

It is the process whereby electrical impulses are used to identify the problem/condition, existing in a muscle, nerve or both. Thereby helps in analysis by methods of recording, display and measurement.

Electrical impulses are used for the diagnostic purpose.

Current used: Interrupted direct current

Types of electrodiagnostic tests in interest of physioytherapist are:

1. Strength duration curve (SDC)
2. Nerve conduction velocity test (NCVT)
3. Electromyography (EMG)

Definition

It is the study of electrical activity of a muscle by the way of needle or surface electrodes which are either inserted in or placed over the skin.

This technique consists of observation, analysis and interpretation of electrical activity of muscles or nerves, so also known as electroneuromyography (ENMG) and the instrument used for the technique is called electromyograph and the produces record is called electromyogram.

Uses

Diagnosis of conditions like
- Spinal muscular atrophy
- Syringomyelia
- Poliomyelitis
- Post-polio syndrome
- Inflammatory muscle disease like
  ↳ Polymyositis
  ↳ Viral myositis
- Myopathies like
  ↳ Metabolic myopathies
  ↳ Congenital myopathies
  ↳ Myotonic dystrophy
- Dystrophies like
  ↳ Duchenne muscular dystrophy
  ↳ Becker muscular dystrophy
  ↳ Limb girdle muscular dystrophy
  ↳ Myotonic dystrophy
  ↳ Facioscapulohumeral muscular dystrophy
- Lesions of anterior horn cells
- Lesions of nerves and muscles

Apparatus

1. Electrodes
   - Needle
     a. Concentric
     b. Monopolar
     c. Single fiber
     d. Macro-needle
   - Surface electrodes are in the form of disk, cup, ring
2. EMG unit
3. Filters
4. Amplifier
5. Display unit
6. Averager
7. Cotton swab
8. Spirit

Guidelines

Apparatus Preparation

- Check for any cut, break in the power cable.
- Prepare procedure trolly with cotton swabs.

Patient Preparation

- Clean the skin with cotton swab soaked in spirit.
- Select the electrode and place it over the desired area.

  Note: Knowledge of muscle anatomy is a must to perform this procedure.

Techniques

a. Surface EMG

- Records muscle activity from the surface of the muscle underlying the skin.
- Provide only a limited assessment of the muscle activity.

Limitations:

- Recordings are restricted to superficial muscles.
- Fatty patients have weaker emg signals.

b. Intermuscular EMG

- Simple approach is by a monopolar needle electrode.
- Fine wire inserted into a muscle with a surface electrode as a reference or two fine wires inserted into muscle referenced to each other.

Use:

- For research or kinesiology studies.
- To see maximum muscle contraction
- To indicate amount of muscle fatigue.

  Diagnostic monopolar EMG electrodes are stiff so that these can penetrate the skin and are insulated, with its tip exposed using a surface electrode for reference.

Concentric Needle Electrode

- Complex in design.
- Made of fine wire, insulated. Shaft is exposed and serve as the reference electrode.
- Exposed tip of the fine wire serves as the active electrode.

Advantage

- Small signals
- Reduced electrical artifacts from tissue.
- Reliable measures.

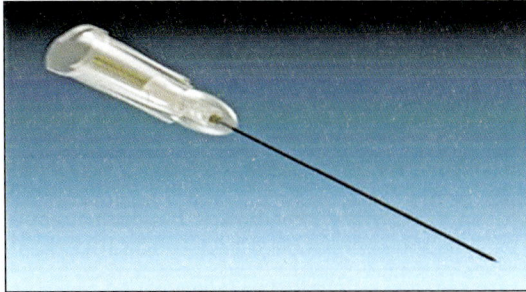

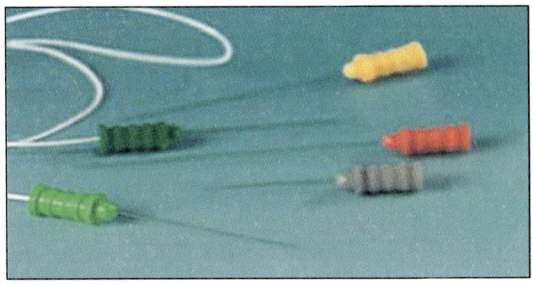

Monopolar Needle

Procedure

1. Patient skin preparation is done.
2. Monopolar or concentric needle electrode is inserted through the skin into the muscular tissue.
3. Needle is then moved to multiple spots in a relaxed muscle and to insertional and resting activity of the muscle are evaluated.
4. Normal muscles exhibit a brief burst of muscle fiber activity which lasts for 100 ms.

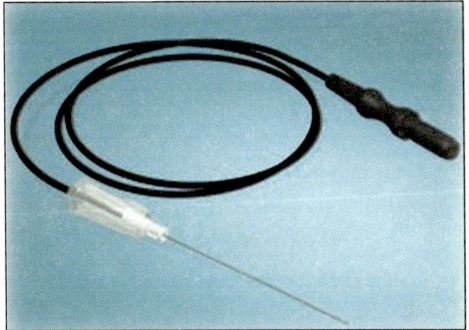

5. Resting and insertional activities are evaluated by the electromyographer.
6. Activity is analyzed by retracting the electrode few millimetres and is repeated.
7. Due to difference in the internal structure of skeletal muscle, the electrode is placed at

several points so that an accurate study can be performed.

Contraindications

- Pacemakers
- Lymphoedema
- Cellulitis

Limitation

It is less informative for patients who are:
- Not willing or not co-operative
- Children and infants
- Paralytic patients
- Obesity

CT Scan (Computerised Tomography Scan)

It is a scan that combines a series of X-ray images taken from different angles and uses computer processing to create cross-sectional images, or slices, of the bones, blood vessels and soft tissues inside your body.

CT scan images provide more detailed information than plain X-rays do.

- It is used to quickly examine people who may have internal injuries from car accidents or other types of trauma.
- It can be used to visualize nearly all parts of the body.
- It is used to diagnose disease or injury as well as to plan medical, surgical or radiation treatment.

Procedure

- The patient should lie on a narrow table that slides into the center of the CT scanner.
- Inside the machine, the X-ray beam rotates around the body while the modern spiral scanner can perform exam without stopping.

- A computer creates separate images of the body area, called slices.
- These images can be stored, viewed on a monitor, or printed on film.
- Three-dimensional models of the body area can be created by stacking the slices together.
- The patient should stay still during the procedure otherwise slight movement can cause a blurred image.
- The patient has to hold the breath for short periods of time during the procedure.
- Complete scans most often take only a few minutes.
- The newest scanners can image your entire body in less than 30 seconds.

Test Preparations

- A special dye called contrast is to be delivered into the body before the test starts. Contrast helps certain areas show up better on the X-rays.
- If the patient has any type of allergy to contrast then the doctors prescribed medicine prior to the test in order to avoid any other reaction.

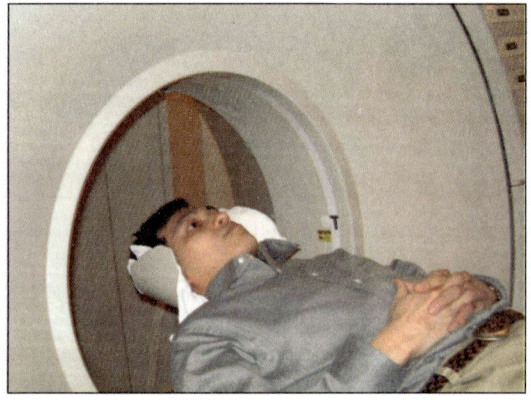

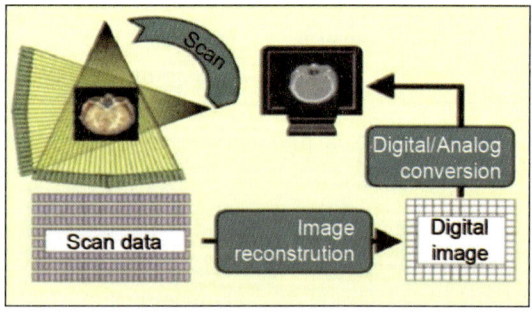

3 steps of CT imaging

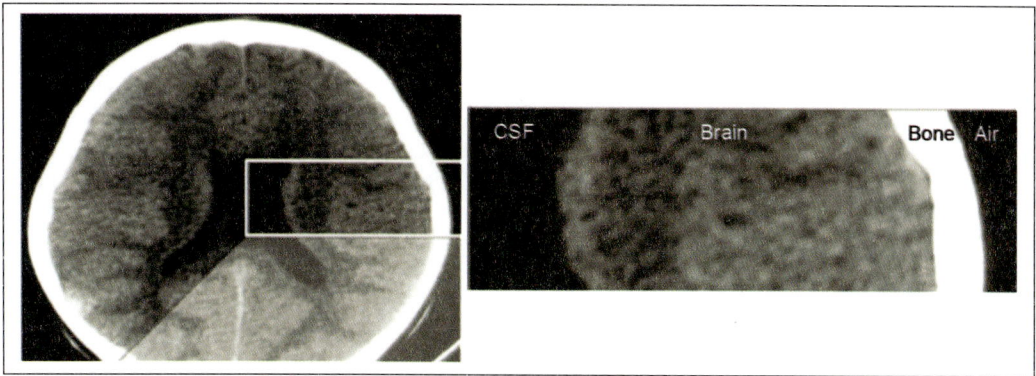

Densities on CT scan

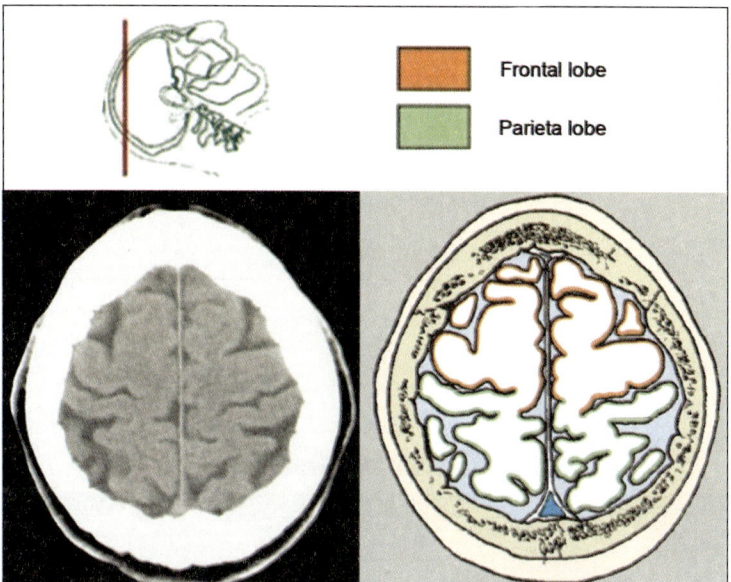

Sections showing lobes

- Contrast can be given several ways, depending on the type of CT being performed. It may be delivered through a vein (IV) in hand or forearm or into the rectum using an enema.

- Prior to the test, the patient has to drink the contrast which depends on the type of exam being done. It may taste chalky, although some are flavoured. The contrast passes out of the body through stools.

- If contrast is used, the patient is asked not to drink or eat anything for 4 to 6 hours prior to the test.

- Prior to the test, the patient is asked to wear a hospital gown with all the metal things form the body, e.g. jewellery, hair pins, safety pins, etc. should be removed.

Physiological Effects

- Some people may have discomfort from lying on the hard table.

- Contrast given through an IV may cause a slight burning feeling, a metallic taste in the mouth, and a warm flushing of the body. These sensations are normal and usually go away within a few seconds.

Indication

- A CT scan creates detailed pictures of the body, including the brain, chest, spine, and abdomen.
- Diagnose an infection.
- Guide a surgeon to the right area during a biopsy.
- Identify masses and tumors, including cancer.
- Study blood vessels.

Risks

Risks of CT scans include:
- Allergic reaction to the contrast dye: The most common type of contrast given into a vein contains iodine. If you have an iodine allergy, a type of contrast may cause nausea or vomiting, sneezing, itching, or hives.
- Damage to kidney function from the contrast dye

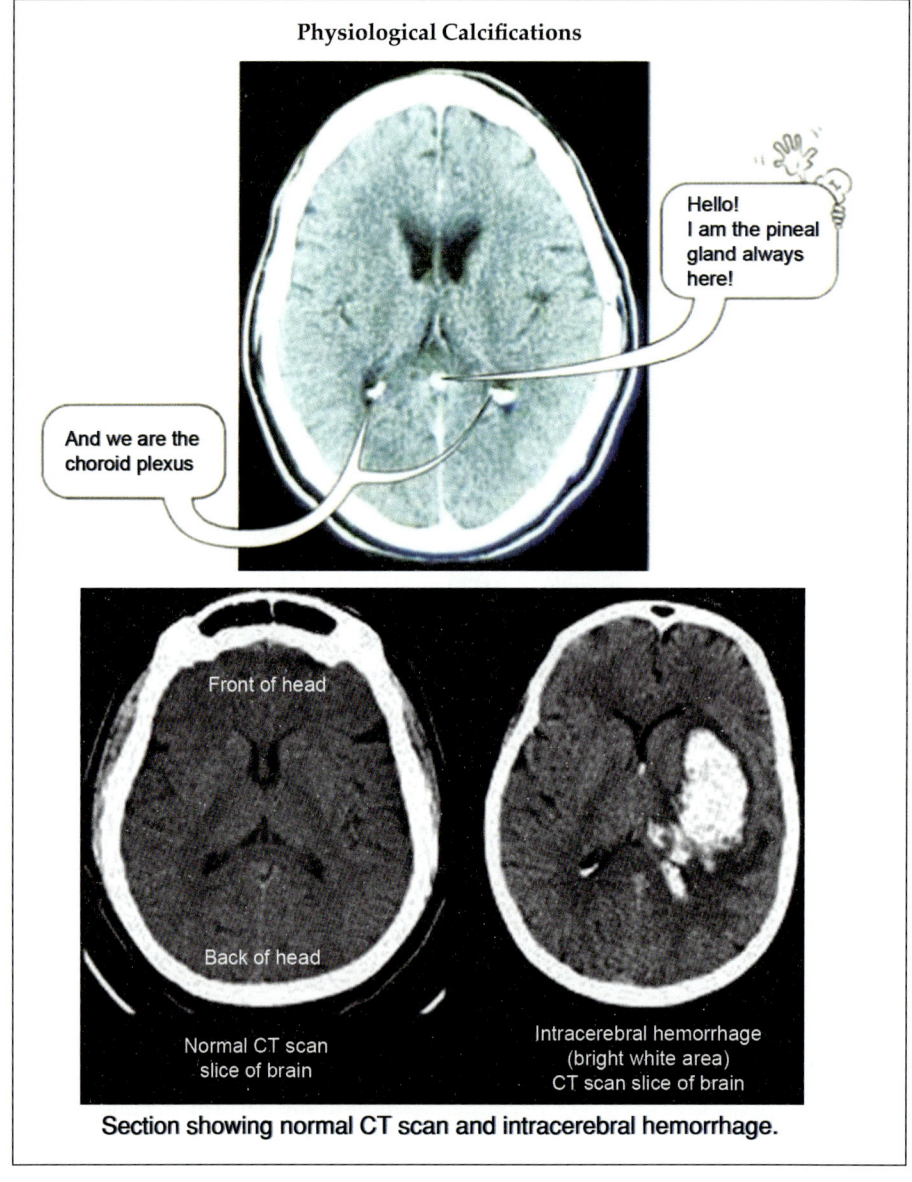

Section showing normal CT scan and intracerebral hemorrhage.

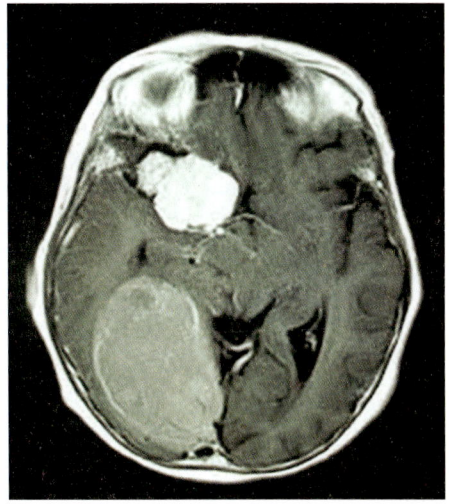

CT scan tumour

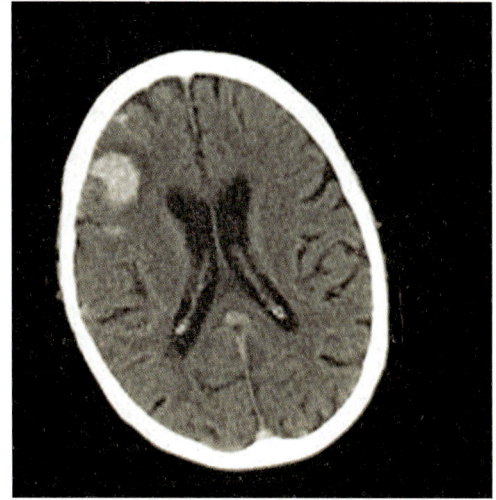

CT scan concussion

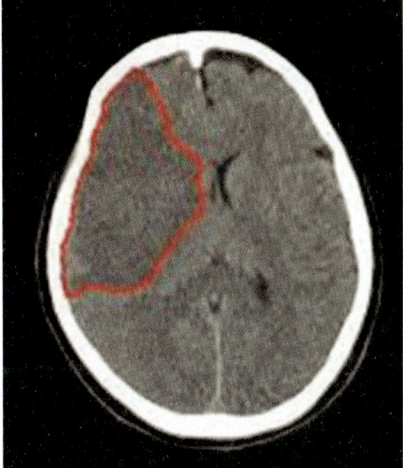

CT scan stroke

- Exposure to radiation
  Having many X-rays or CT scans over time may increase your risk for cancer

Alternative Names

CAT scan; computed axial tomography scan; computed tomography scan.

Magnetic Resonance Imaging (MRI)

The magnetic resonance imaging is used in radiology to investigate the anatomy and physiology of the body in both health and disease.

It uses a powerful magnetic field known as radio waves to produce detailed pictures of the body's internal structures that are clearer to identify and accurately characterize disease than other imaging methods.

It is used to examine the body for various diseases including tumors and diseases of the liver, heart, and bowel.

It may also be used to monitor an unborn child in the womb.

MRI is non-invasive and does not use ionizing radiation.

MR imaging of the body is performed to evaluate:
• Organs of the trunk like heart, liver, biliary tract, kidneys, spleen, bowel, pancreas, and adrenal glands.

• Pelvic organs including the bladder and the reproductive organs such as the uterus and ovaries in females and the prostate gland in males.
• Blood vessels (including MR angiography).
• Lymph nodes.

The physicians use an MR examination to diagnose or monitor treatment for conditions such as:

• Malformations of the blood vessels and inflammation of the vessels.
• Tumors of the chest, abdomen or pelvis.
• Fetus in the womb of a pregnant woman.
• Diseases of the liver, such as cirrhosis, and abnormalities of the bile ducts and pancreas.
• Inflammatory bowel disease such as ulcerative colitis.
• Heart problems, such as congenital heart disease.

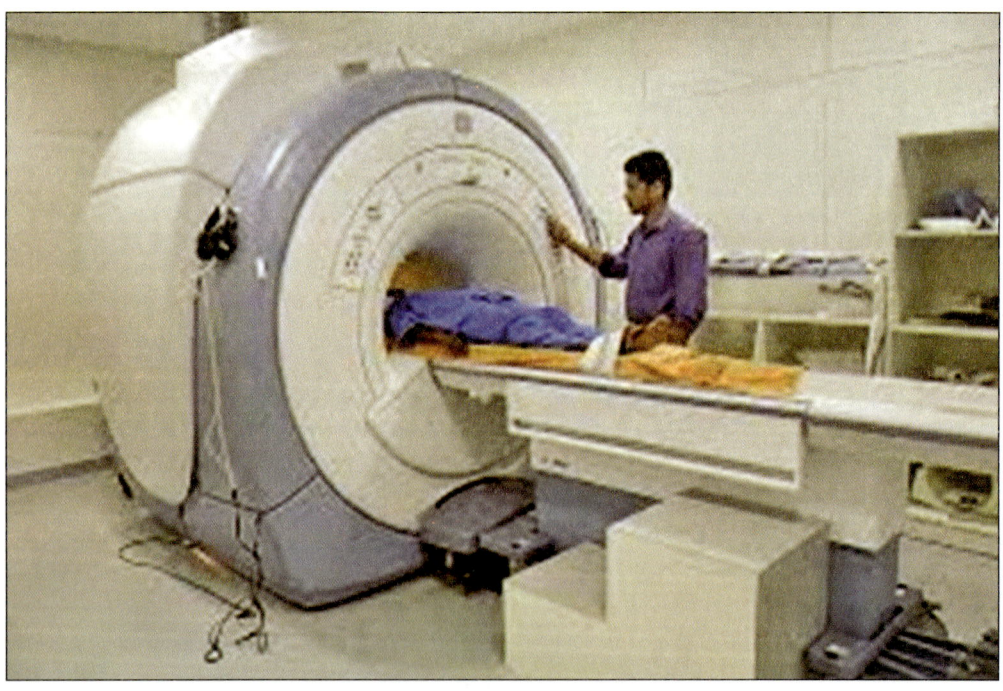

Procedure

- The patient should wear a gown or their own loose fitting with non-metal fastener clothing.
- Place the patient on a movable examination table and with the help of straps and bolsters the patient maintain the still and correct position during imaging.
- MRI examinations may be performed on outpatients or inpatients.
- Devices that contain coils capable of sending and receiving radio waves may be placed around or adjacent to the area of the body being studied.
- If a contrast material has been used in the MRI exam, there will be a insertion of intravenous catheter, also known as an IV line, vein or arm of a patient.
- A saline solution may be used to inject the contrast material.
- The solution will drip through the IV to prevent blockage of the IV catheter until the contrast material is injected.
- Prior to MRI, an injection of contrast material gadolinium can be used in patients with iodine contrast allergy, but may require pre-medication injected into the bloodstream.
- Later intravenous line will be removed.

- The radiologist must ask for any allergies such as an allergy to iodine or X-ray contrast material, drugs, food, or the environment, or if you have asthma or to any serious health issues such as recent surgeries, for severe kidney disease, it will be necessary to perform a blood test to determine whether the kidneys are functioning adequately.
- The pregnant women should not have this exam in the first trimester of pregnancy.
- If patient has fear of enclosed spaces or anxiety, a mild sedative prior to the examination is needed.
- Jewelry and other accessories such as hair pin, credit cards, hearing aids, zipper, eyeglasses, etc. should be left at home if possible, or removed prior to the MRI scan. Because they can interfere with the magnetic field of the MRI unit.
- An MRI exam is safe for patients with metal implants, except for a few types. People with the following implants cannot be scanned and should not enter the MRI scanning area.
  - ✎ Nearly all cardiac defibrillators and pacemakers.
  - ✎ Cochlear (ear) implant.
  - ✎ Some types of clip used for brain aneurysms.
  - ✎ Some types of metal coil placed within blood vessels.

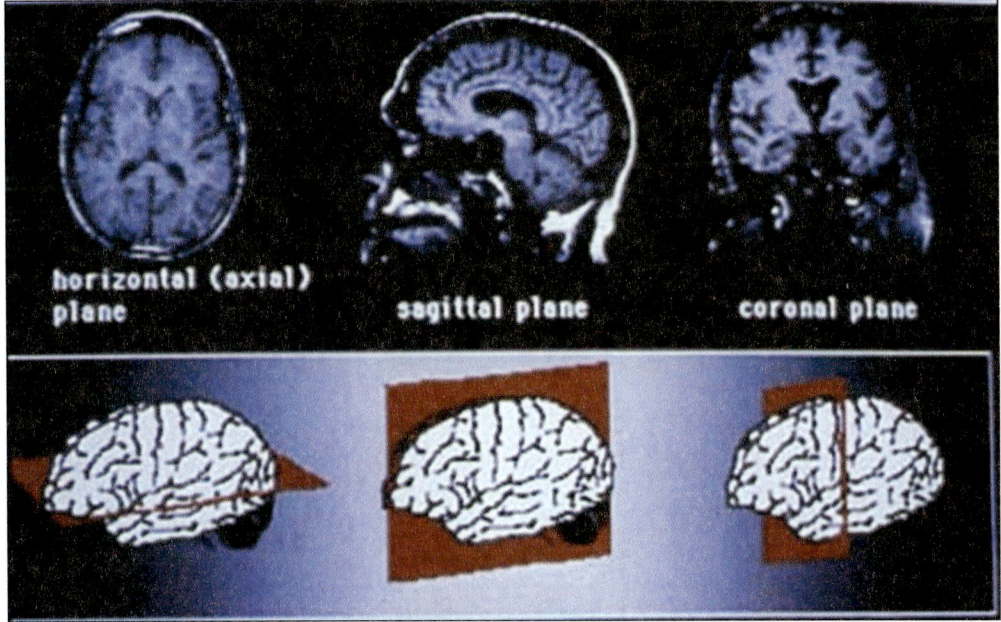

MRI—3 planar view

- Prior to the investigation, it is the patient responsibility to tell about any medical or electronic devices incorporate his/her into body.
  - ♴ Artificial heart valves
  - ♴ Implanted drug infusion ports

- ♴ Artificial limbs or metallic joint prostheses
- ♴ Implanted nerve stimulators.
- Depending on the type of exam and the equipment used, the entire exam is usually completed in 30 to 50 minutes.

Construction and Working

It is a large cylinder-shaped tube surrounded which is designed in a fashion that the magnet does not completely surround the patient by a circular magnet.

Unlike conventional X-ray examinations and computed tomography (CT) scans, magnetic resonance imaging does not utilize an ionizing radiation. Instead, radio waves redirect alignment of hydrogen atoms that naturally exist within the body without causing any chemical changes in the tissues. As the hydrogen atoms return to their usual alignment, they emit energy that varies according to the type of body tissue from which they come. The MR scanner captures this energy and creates a picture of the tissues scanned based on the information, then the magnetic field is produced by flowing electric current through wire coils, other coils, located in the machine and in some cases, placed around

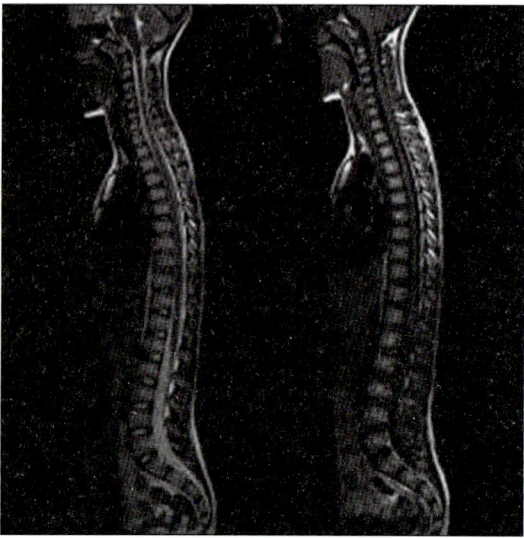

Full length spine
(normal MRI appearance)

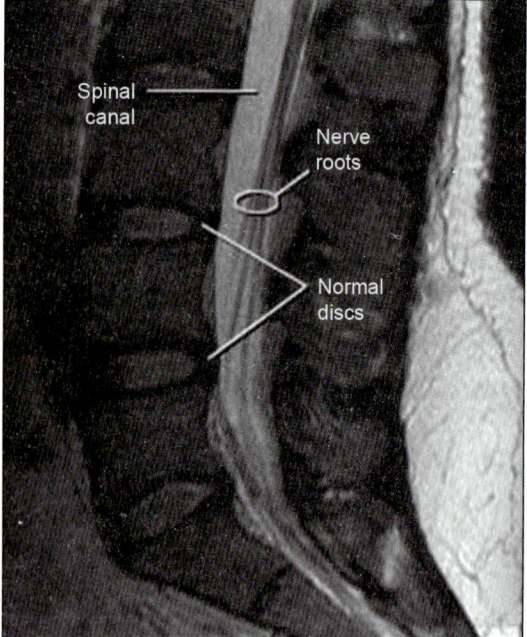

Normal lumbar spine

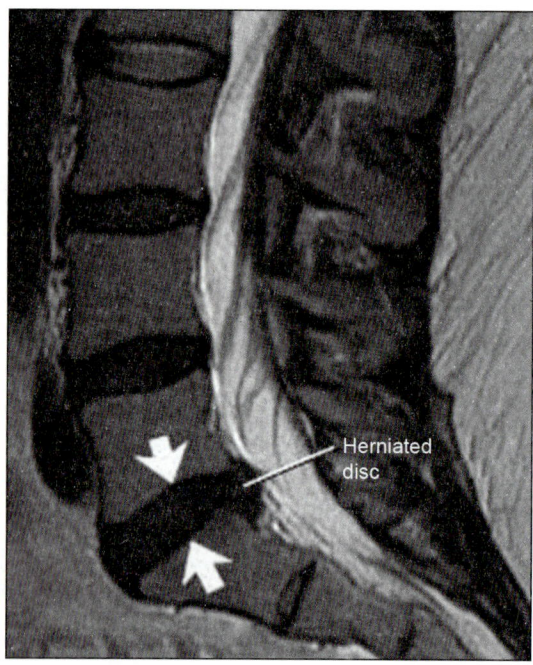

Herniated disc of lumbar spine

the part of the body being imaged, send and receive radio waves, producing signals that are detected by the coils, then the computer processes and generates a series of images showing a thin slice of the body that studied from different angles for interpretation of a radiologist/physician.

Side Effects
- Most MRI exams are painless.
- Some patients find it uncomfortable to remain still during MR imaging.
- Others experience a sense of being closed-in (claustrophobia). Therefore, sedation can be arranged for those patients who anticipate anxiety, but fewer than one in 20 require medication.

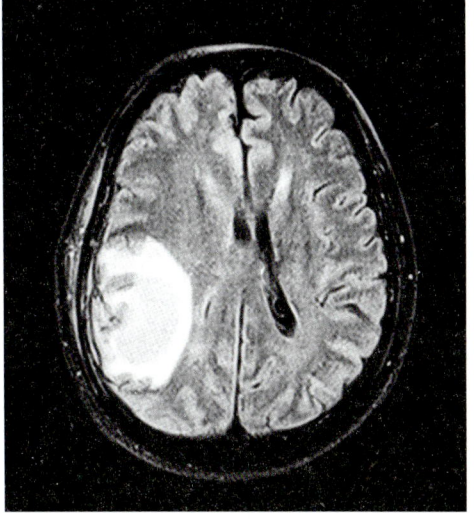

MRI brain: Showing brain tumor at right parietal lobe of cerebrum

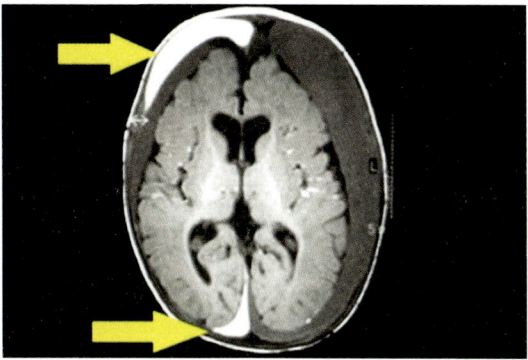

MRI shows bilateral fluid collections as a result of chronic bilateral subdural hematomas and new subdural hematomas in the right frontal and posterior interhemispheric region. The bright signal is a result of methemoglobin indicating subacute hematoma (about one week old).

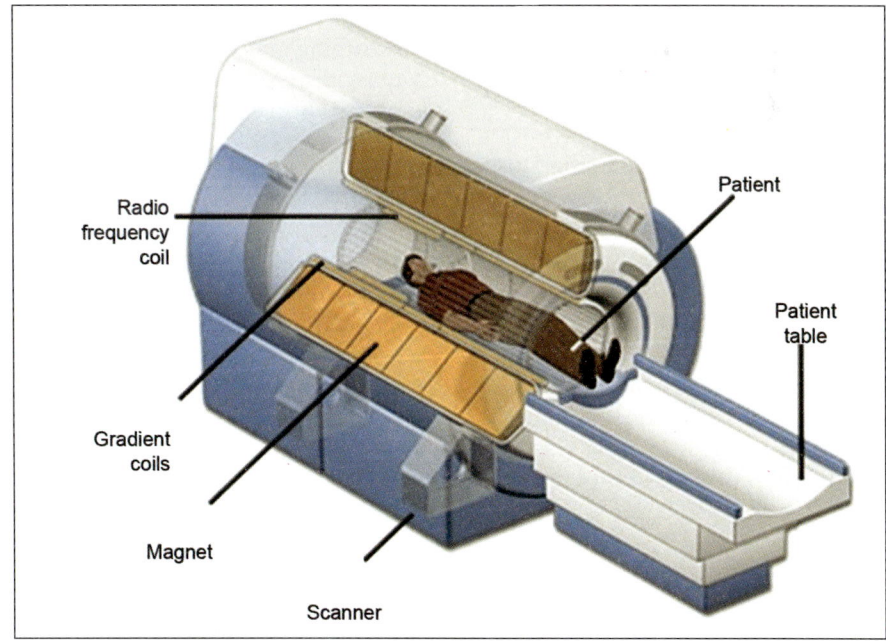

MRI scanner cutaway

- Children will be given appropriately sized earplugs or headphones during the exam. Music may be played through the headphones to help you pass the time.
- Sometimes the intravenous needle may cause discomfort when it is inserted while some experience some bruising.
- There is also a very small chance of irritation of skin at the site of the IV tube insertion.
- Some patients may sense a temporary metallic taste in their mouth after the contrast injection.
- On very rare occasions, a few patients experience side effects from the contrast material, including nausea and local pain.
- Similarly, patients are very rarely allergic to the contrast material and experience hives, itchy eyes or other reactions.
- If patients experience allergic symptoms, then immediately notify the technologist.

Benefits

- MRI is a non-invasive imaging technique that does not involve exposure to ionizing radiation.
- MRI produces images of the soft-tissue structures of the body such as the heart, liver and many other organs.
- Identifies and accurately characterize diseases than other imaging methods. This detail makes MRI an invaluable tool in early diagnosis and evaluation of many focal lesions and tumors.
- MRI has proven to be valuable in diagnosing a broad range of conditions, including cancer, heart and vascular diseases, muscular and bone abnormalities.
- MRI allows physicians to assess the biliary system non-invasively and without contrast injection.
- The contrast material used in MRI exams is less likely to produce an allergic reaction than the iodine-based contrast materials used for conventional X-rays and CT scanning.

- MRI provides a non-invasive alternative to X-ray, angiography and CT for diagnosing problems of the heart and blood vessels.

Risks

- The MRI examination poses almost no risk to the average patient when appropriate safety guidelines are followed.
- There is a very slight risk of an allergic reaction, if contrast material is injected. Such reactions usually are mild and easily controlled by medication.
- If sedation is used, there are risks of excessive sedation. However, the technologist or nurse monitors your vital signs to minimize this risk.
- Although the strong magnetic field is not harmful in itself, implanted medical devices that contain metal may malfunction or cause problems during an MRI exam.

Limitation

- The tall-sized patients may not fit into the opening of certain types of MRI machines.
- The presence of an implant or other metallic object sometimes makes it difficult to obtain clear images. Patient movement can have the same effect.
- Irregular heart beat may affect the quality of images.
- Breathing may cause artifacts, or image distortions, during MRIs of the chest, abdomen and pelvis. Bowel motion is another source of motion artifacts in abdomen and pelvic MRI studies. This is less of a problem with state-of-the art scanners and techniques.
- Although there is no reason to believe that magnetic resonance imaging harms the fetus, pregnant women usually are advised not to have an MRI exam during the first trimester unless medically necessary or advised.
- MRI may not always distinguish between cancer tissue and fluid, known as edema.
- MRI typically costs more and may take more time to perform than other imaging modalities

How to Check the BMI (Body Mass Index)?

Apparatus required: Pencil, paper, inchtape, bathroom scale, caluculator.

Procedure

1. First check the weight of the person without shoes
2. Check the height of the patient
3. Now caluculate the BMI based on the following formula and report

   BMI = Weight (kg)/[Height (m) × Height (m)]

Result

The desirable BMI range for adult (aged 18 and above) is between 18.5 and 25.
- If your BMI is less than 18.5, you are underweight
- If your BMI is 18.5 to less than 25, your weight is desirable.

- If your BMI is 25 to less than 30, you are overweight.
- If your BMI is 30 or more, you are obese.

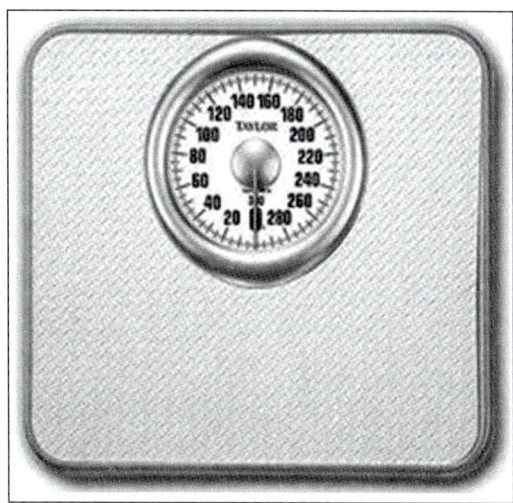

Bathroom scale

Manual Muscle Testing

INDIVIDUAL MUSCLE TESTING

The manual muscle testing is the numerical value that ranges from '0' which means no response to '5' that means best response. The manual muscle testing comprises of 2 factors:

a. Subjective factor
b. Objective factor

Subjective factor: The amount of resistance given prior to the actual test and the amount that the patient tolerates during the testing procedure.

Objective factor: It is the patient's ability to perform activities according to the grading system of MMT, e.g. '0' means no contraction so patient won't be able to perform any movement or contractions according to the criteria of grading system.

GRADING SYSTEM

Numerical score	Test performance/qualitative score
5	Normal (N)
4	Good (G)
3	Fair (F)
2	Poor (P)
1	Trace activity (T)
0	Zero (no activity) (())

Test

a. **The break test:** If the subject is asked to move the limb to its end range and when that position is reached, the examiner applies manual resistance to break the hold and applies force in opposite direction. This process is called as break test and is most commonly used for practising MMT.

b. **Active resistance test:** It is an application of manual resistance against an actively contracting muscle or muscle group.

CRITERIA FOR ASSIGNING A MUSCLE TEST GRADE

Grade 5 (normal)	Grade 4 (good)	Grade 3 (fair)	Grade 2 (poor)	Grade 1 (trace)	Grade 0 (no activity)
a. When the examiner cannot break the hold position of patient then grade 5 is assigned.	a. When examiner can break the hold position of patient then grade 4 is assigned.	a. Muscle can move against resistance but when applying even a mild resistance causes motion to break, the muscle is assigned as grade 3.	a. Movement in gravity eliminated position is grade 2	a. When examiner can only visualize or palpate some contractile activity in muscle or feel a tendon popping up during movement then grade 1 is assigned	a. When not even a traces of activity is felt then grade 0 is assigned
b. Normal muscle performance	b. True weakness	b. Full range of motion against gravity but with no resistance.	b. Poor muscle response.	b. No movement only traces contractile activity	b. No activity, no contraction

	Grade scale 5–0	
0	None/no acitivity	No visible or palpable contraction
1	Trace	Visible or palpable contraction with no motion.
2	Poor	Full range of motion with gravity eliminated position.
3	Fair	Full range of motion against gravity
4	Good	Full range of motion against gravity with moderate resistance.
5	Normal	Full range of motion against gravity with maximal resistance

PREPARATION FOR THE MUSCLE TESTING

1. A patient should be free from all discomfort or pain during testing procedures.
2. The environment should be quiet and comfortable with no distractions, etc.
3. There should be a firm plinth or mat table so that stabilization becomes easy.
4. There should be adequate stabilization of the part to be tested.
5. Materials needed are:
   a. Documentation form of muscle testing
   b. Pillows, towel for positioning
   c. Pen, pencil
   d. Sheets or linens.
   e. Assistance for stabilization, turning or moving the patient.

MUSCLE TESTING—UPPER EXTREMITY

Testing muscles of part		Muscle	Testing muscles of part		Muscle
Shoulder			2	Extension	Extensor carpi radialis longus, extensor carpi ulnaris and extensor carpi radialis brevis
1	Flexion	Anterior deltoid and coraco-brachialis			
2	Extension	Latissimus dorsi, teres major, posterior deltoid.	**Finger**		
3	Abduction	Middle deltoid and supras-pinatus	1	MP flexion	Lumbricals and interossei
			2	PIP and DIP flexion	Flexor digitorum superficialis and flexor digitorum pro-fundus
4	Adduction	Pectoralis major.			
5	External rotation	Infraspinatus and teres minor.	3	MP extension	Extensor digitorum and indices
6	Internal rotation	Subscapularis.	4	Finger abduction	Dorsal interossei
Elbow			5	Finger adduction	Palmar interossei
1	Flexion	Biceps brachialis, brachioradialis	6	Thumb MP and IP flexion	Flexor policis brevis and longus
2	Extension	Triceps brachii	7	Thumb MP and IP extension	Extensor policis brevis and longus
Forearm					
1	Supination	Supinator and biceps brachii	8	Thumb abduction	Abductor pollicis longus and brevis
2	Pronation	Pronator teres and pronator quadratus	9	Thumb adduction	Adductor pollicis
Wrist			10	Opposition	Opponens pollicis and opponens digiti minimi
1	Flexion	Flexor carpi radialis and flexor carpi ulnaris			

Shoulder Flexion Grades 4 and 5

Patient position	Therapist position	Testing/procedure	Instruction	Result
Short sitting position, slight elbow flexion, forearm pronated	Stand at test side. One hand giving resistance to the distal humerus above elbow and other hand stabilize the shoulder.	Shoulder flexion 90° without rota-tion with abduction and upward rota-tion of scapula.	Raise your arm at shoulder level. Hold it. Don't let me push it down	Grade 5: Hold end position against maximal resistance. Grade 4: Hold end position against moderate resistance.

Shoulder Flexion Grade 3

Same as above	Stand at the test side	Patient flexes shoulder at 90°	Raise your arm forward to shoulder side.	Full range without resistance.

Shoulder Flexion Grades 2, 1 and 0

Same as above	Stand at test side. Palpate over the superior and anterior surface of deltoid muscle.	Attempt to flex shoulder to 90°	Raise your arm Try it	Grade 2: Complete partial ROM against gravity. Grade 1: Feels only contractile activity no movement. Grade 0: No contraction.

Shoulder Extension Grades 4 and 5

Patient position	Therapist position	Testing/procedure	Instruction	Result
Prone lying with head turned to one side.arms at the side, palm up	Stand at the test side. Grasp the both hands over the distal forearm	Patient depresses the arm in down-ward direction	Reach towards your feet Hold it Don't let me push your arm upward towards your head.	Grade 5: Perform full range against maxi-mum resistance Grade 4: Perform full range against mode-rate resistance.

Shoulder Extension Grades 3 and 2

Same as above	Stand at test side	Same as above	Same as above	Grade 3: Perform the available range without resistance. Grade 2: Perform partial range of motion.

Shoulder Extension Grades 1 and 0

Same as above	Stand at test side and palpate below and side of the inferoior angle of scapula.	Attempt to lift arm off the table.	Lift your arm up off the table	Grade 1: No motion only contractile activity Grade 0: No contraction no motion.

Shoulder Abduction Grades 5, 4 and 3

Patient position	Therapist position	Testing/procedure	Instruction	Result
Short sitting, arm at the side.	Stand behind the patient and place your hand above elbow and one hand should stabilize the shoulder girdle.	Patient should ab-duct the arm to 90°.	Raise your arm outside to the shoulder level Hold it Don't let me push it down.	Grade 5: Perform full range against maxi-mum downward resis-tance. Grade 4: Perform full range against moderate downward resistance.

Contd.

Contd.

				Grade 3: Perform the available range to 90° without resistance
Shoulder Abduction Grade 2				
Same as above	Stand behind the patient and palpate the deltoid lateral to the acromion process superiorly	Attempt to abduct the arm	Try to lift your arm outside	*Grade 2*: Perform partial ROM
Shoulder Abduction Grades 1 and 0				
Short sitting	Stand at the side of the patient, shoulder 90° abduction providing limb support at the elbow	Patient tries to maintain arm in abduction.	Try to hold your arm	*Grade 1*: No motion only contraction of deltoid *Grade 0*: No contraction, no motion

Shoulder Adduction Grades 5 and 4				
Patient position	*Therapist position*	*Testing/procedure*	*Instruction*	*Result*
Supine lying with shoulder and elbow abducted to 90°.	Stand at the side of the shoulder. One hand will give resistance just proximal to the wrist and other will check the activity of the pectoralis major muscle just medial to the shoulder joint.	Patient horizontally adduct the shoulder to available ROM.	Move your arm above the chest. Hold it and don't let me push it back	*Grade 5*: Perform full range against maximum resistance. *Grade 4*: Perform full range against moderate resistance
Shoulder Adduction Grade 3				
Same as above	Same as above	Patient horizontally adduct the limb across chest without using diagonal motion.	Same as above without resistance.	*Grade 3*: Perform the available ROM without resistance.
Shoulder Adduction Grades 2, 1 and 0				
Same as above	Same as above	Patient attempts to adduct the shoulder	Move your arm across your chest and try it	*Grade 2*: Patient perform horizontal adduction through available ROM with test arm supported by examiner *Grade 1*: No motion only contraction of pectoralis muscle *Grade 0*: No contraction, no motion.

Shoulder External Rotation Grades 5, 4 and 3				
Patient Position	*Therapist Position*	*Testing/procedure*	*Instruction*	*Result*
Prone lying with head turned to-	Stand at the test side at patient waist level, two	Patient will perform upward	Raise the forearm upward towards	*Grade 5*: Perform full range and holds firmly

Contd.

Contd.

Patient position	Therapist position	Testing/procedure	Instruction	Result
wards the side, shoulder abducted to 90° and is suppor-ted to table, forearm hanging vertically downward, place the towel over the elbow	fingers of one hand will give resistance to wrist and other will support the elbow	movement of the forearm	the table, hold it, don't let me push your hand down	against two finger resistance *Grade 4*: Perform full range but muscles at the end range gives way *Grade 3*: Completes available range of motion without manual resistance

Shoulder External Rotation Grades 2, 1 and 0

Patient position	Therapist position	Testing/procedure	Instruction	Result
Prone lying with head turned to-wards the side, trunk at the edge of the table, the entire limb will hang down loosely with palm facing table.	Sit on a low stool at the shoulder level, palpate the infraspinatus, teres minor on the inferior margin of axilla.	Attempt to exter-nally rotate the shoulder	Turn your palm outward	*Grade 2*: Available range is completed in gravity eliminated position *Grade 1*: No motion only flicker of contraction is seen in both muscles. *Grade 0*: No motion, no contraction.

Shoulder Internal Rotation Grades 5, 4 and 3

Patient position	Therapist position	Testing/procedure	Instruction	Result
Prone lying with head turned to side, shoulder abducted to 90° and is supported on table, place a folded towel over the distal elbow. Forearm is hanging	Stand at the test side. One hand is placed over the volar side of the forearm just above the wrist	Patient moves the arm upward and backward	Move your arm up and back Hold it Do not let me to push it down	*Grade 5*: Perform full range and hold firmly against strong resistance *Grade 4*: Perform full range but a spongy feeling against strong resistance *Grade 3*: Completes available range of motion without manual resistance

Shoulder Internal Rotation Grades 2, 1 and 0

Patient position	Therapist position	Testing/procedure	Instruction	Result
Prone lying, patient near the edge of the table so that arm can hang freely and palm facing towards the table	Stand on the test side and palpate the tendon of subscapularis in the central area of the axilla. Stabilize the test arm at the shoulder	Patient internally rotate the arm with palm facing outward away from the table	Turn your palm inward so that palm facing away from the table	*Grade 2*: Available range is completed in gravity eliminated position *Grade 1*: No motion only flicker of contraction *Grade 0*: No motion, no contraction

Elbow Flexion Grades 5, 4 and 3

Patient position	Therapist position	Testing/procedure	Instruction	Result
Short sitting with arm at the side	Stand towards the test side in front of patient. One hand gives resistance over the pro-	Patient flexes elbow through the available range	Bend your elbow Hold it Do not let me to pull it down	*Grade 5*: Perform full range and holds firmly against strong resistance

Contd.

Contd.

				Grade 4: Perform available range against strong to moderate resistance
				Grade 3: Completes available range of motion without manual resistance
ximal wrist and other hand stabilizes the ant. superior surface of shoulder.				

Elbow Flexion Grades 2, 1 and 0

| Supine lying with elbow flexed to 45° with forearm supinated for bicep, pronated for brachialis and in mid-prone position for brachioradialis | Stand at the test side in front of patient and support the arm and wrist, palpate the bicep in anticubital fossa, brachialis in distal arm and brachioradialis on the proximal volar surface of forearm | Patient attempt to flex the elbow | Bend your elbow (try it) | Grade 2: Available range is completed in gravity eliminated position. Grade 1: Examiner can palpate these three muscles contractile response. Grade 0: No palpable contraction. |

Elbow Extension Grades 5, 4 and 3

Patient position	*Therapist position*	*Testing/procedure*	*Instruction*	*Result*
Prone lying with shoulder abducted 90° with arm hanging vertically from the side of the table	Stand at the test side, one hand hold the arm above the elbow and the other give downward resistance distal to the forearm on the dorsal surface	Patient should extend the elbow to the available range	Straighten your elbow Hold it Do not let me to pull it down	Grade 5: Perform full range and holds firmly against strong resistance Grade 4: Perform available range against strong to moderate resistance Grade 3: Completes available range of motion without manual resistance

Elbow Extension Grades 2, 1 and 0

| Short sitting with shoulder abducted 90° and in neutral position with elbow flexed to 45°. The limb is horizontal to floor | Stand at the test side for grade 2 support the limb at the elbow and for grade 1 and 0 support it under the forearm 7 palpate the tendon tricep muscle. | Patient should attempt to extend the elbow | Straighten your elbow (try it) | Grade 2: Available range is completed in gravity eliminated position Grade 1: Examiner can palpate the muscles contractile response Grade 0: No palpable contraction |

Wrist Flexion Grades 5 and 4

Patient position	*Therapist position*	*Testing/procedure*	*Instruction*	*Result*
Short sitting forearm supported on the table. Forearm is supinated with	Distal forearm is supported under the wrist	Patient should flex the wrist keeping the digits and fingers relaxed	Bend your wrist Hold it Do not let me to pull it down	Grade 5: Perform full range with flexion and holds against strong resistance

Contd.

Contd.

wrist in neutral position				Grade 4: Perform available range against strong to moderate resistance

Wrist Flexion Grade 3

Starting position with forearm supinated and wrist is in neutral position	Support patient forearm under the wrist area	Patient flexes the wrist without giving resistance.	Bend your wrist Keep your finger relaxed and straight.	Grade 3: Completes available range without manual resistance.

Wrist Flexion Grade 2

Short sitting with forearm supported on table and hand resting on ulnar side	Patient forearm is supported proximal to the wrist	Patient flexes the wrist from the ulnar side. Hold the distal forearm so that the forearm not lie on to the table and ask the patient to do flexion motion	Bend your wrist and keep your finger in a relaxed state	Grade 2: Available range is completed without gravity assis-tance.

Wrist Flexion Grades 1 and 0

The forearm is supinated and is supported on the table	The wrist is supported in flexion position and using the other hand palpate the tendon (flexor carpi radialis, flexor carpi ulnaris).	Patient will attempt to flex the elbow	Bend your wrist (try it)	Grade 1: Examiner can palpate the tendon of these two muscles contractile response Grade 0: No palpable contraction

Wrist Extension Grades 5, 4 and 3

Patient position	Therapist position	Testing/procedure	Instruction	Result
Short sitting position with forearm is fully pronated, elbow is flexed and this position is supported on to the table	Stand at the test side and support the distal forearm and other hand gives resistance onto the dorsal surface of the metacarpals	Patient should extend the wrist only not the fingers	Pull your wrist up and do not let me to push it down	Grade 5: Perform full range with extension and holds against strong resistance
	For extensor carpi radialis longus and brevis, resistance is given on to the 2nd and 3rd metacarpals.			Grade 4: Perform available range against strong to moderate resistance
	For extensor carpi ulnaris, the resistance is given on to the dorsal surface of the 5th metacarpal			Grade 3: Perform full range

Wrist Extension Grade 2

The forearm is in neutral position and is supported on the table	Patient wrist is grapsed so that hand should not touch the table	Patient extend the wrist	The wrist should be bend back	Grade 2: Available range is completed with gravity eliminated.

Contd.

Contd.

Wrist Extension Grade 1 and 0				
The hand fully pronated and is supported on the table with forearm	The patient wrist is supported in extension. With the other hand palpate the tendon using one finger	The patient will attempt to extend the wrist	Bring your wrist back (try it)	*Grade 1*: Examiner can palpate the tendon of the muscle (contractile response). *Grade 0*: No palpable contraction.

MUSCLE TESTING—LOWER EXTREMITY

	Testing muscles of part	*Muscle*
		HIP
1	Flexion	Psoas major, Iliacus, etc.
2	Extension	Gluteus maximus and hamstring
3	Abduction	Gluteus medius and minimus
4	Adduction	Adductor magnus, brevis, longus, etc.
5	External rotation	Obturator internus, externus, piriformis, etc.
6	Internal rotation	Tensor fascia latae, gluteus maximus and medius
		KNEE
1	Flexion	Hamstring
2	Extension	Quadricep femoris
		ANKLE
1	Plantar flexion	Gastrocnemius and soleus
2	Dorsiflexion	Tibialis anterior
		FOOT
1	Inversion	Tibialis posterior
2	Eversion	Peroneus longus and brevis

Hip Flexion Grades 5, 4 and 3				
Patient position	*Therapist position*	*Testing/procedure*	*Instructions*	*Result*
The patient should be in short sitting postion with thigh supported on the table, knee flexed and is hanging vertically and trunk stability is maintainted by placing both the hands on to the sides of couch	Stand at the test side with hand giving resistance to the distal thigh just above the knee	Patient will flex the hip and therapist gives resistance in the downward direction	Lift the leg up-ward, do not let me push it down	*Grade 5*: Perform full range and holds against strong resistance *Grade 4*: Perform available range against strong to moderate resis-tance *Grade 3*: Perform full range and hold the postion without resistance

Hip Flexion Grade 2				
Side lying position, the test limb should be up and is supported by examiner and the lower most limb should be flexed slightly	Stand behind the limb and cradle the test limb in one arm supporting under the knee and other will maintain the trunk alignment	Patient flexes the supported hip	Knee should touch your chest (bring it up to the chest)	*Grade 2:* Available range is completed in side lying posi-tion.

Contd.

Contd.

Hip Flexion Grades 1 and 0

Supine lying position with the test limb supported under the calf with hand of the examiner behind the knee	Stand at the test side with the limb supported under the calf by the hand of examiner behind the knee with the other hand palpate the muscle just medial to the side of the sartorius	Patient attempt to flex the hip	Bring your knee towards your chest try to touch it to your nose	*Grade 1*: Examiner can palpate the tendon of the muscle (contractile response) *Grade 0*: No palpable contraction.

Hip Extension Grades 5, 4 and 3

Patient position	*Therapist position*	*Testing/procedure*	*Instruction*	*Result*
Prone lying position	Stand at the test side at the level of pelvis	Patient extend the hip and examiner resist it in downward direction	Lift your leg without bending your knees Hold it Do not let me push it down	*Grade 5*: Perform full range and holds against strong resistance *Grade 4*: Perform available range against strong to moderate resistance *Grade 3*: Perform full range and hold the postion without resistance

Hip Extension Grade 2

Side lying positon with the test limb supported by examiner and lower limb is flexed slightly	Stand behind the thigh level and the test limb is supported below knee cradling the leg, other hand maintains the hip alignment	Extension of hip through full range of motion	Without bending your knee bring your leg back towards me.	*Grade 2* Available range is completed in side lying position

Hip Extension Grades 1 and 0

Prone lying position	Stand on to the test side at the hip level and palpate the hamstring or gluteus maximus muscle	The patient attempt to extend the hip in prone lying position.	Squeeze your buttocks together.	*Grade 1*: Examiner can palpate hamstring or gluteus maximus muscle (contractile response) but no joint movement is visible *Grade 0*: No palpable contraction. No movement

Hip Abduction Grades 5, 4 and 3

Patient position	*Therapist position*	*Testing/procedure*	*Instruction*	*Result*
Side lying positon with test leg uppermost and lower leg is flexed for stability	Stand behind the patient. One hand gives resistance lateral side of the	Patient abduct the hip without flexing the hip or knee	Lift your test leg up Hold it	*Grade 5*: Perform full range and holds against strong resistance

Contd.

Contd.

	knee in downward direction and other hand palpates the gluteus muscle.		Do not let me push it down	*Grade 4:* Perform available range against strong to moderate resistance
				Grade 3: Perform full range and hold the postion without resistance

Hip Abduction Grade 2

Supine lying	Stand on to the test side. Hold the leg distally under the ankle just to reduce friction, no resistance or assistance is offered during this process.	Patient abducts the hip through the available range	Bring your leg outside the couch	*Grade 2:* Available range is completed in side lying position

Hip Abduction Grades 1 and 0

Supine lying	Stand on to the test side at thigh level with one hand holding the leg distally under the ankle, no resistance or assistance is offered during this process	Patient attempt to abduct the hip	Bring your leg outside the couch (try it)	*Grade 1:* Examiner can palpate gluteus medius muscle (contractile response) but no joint movement is visible *Grade 0:* No palpable contraction. No movement

Hip Adduction Grades 5, 4 and 3

Patient position	*Therapist position*	*Testing/procedure*	*Instruction*	*Result*
Side lying position with test limb supported by table and upper most part is supported (cradling the leg with forearm) by examiner with 25° of abduction	Stand behind knee level with one hand giving resistance to the test limb (lowermost limb) and other cradle the leg (uppermost limb) with the forearm	Patient adduct the hip until the lowermost limb contracts the uppermost limb	Lift your bottom leg up to the top leg	*Grade 5:* Perform full range and holds against strong resistance *Grade 4:* Perform available range against strong to moderate resistance *Grade 3:* Perform full range and hold the postion without resistance

Hip Adduction Grade 2

Supine lying position	Stand at the side of the test limb at the thigh level. One hand will palpate the muscle and other	Patient adduct hip	Bring your leg towards the other leg	*Grade 2:* Available range is completed

Contd.

Contd.

	will hold the limb distally under the ankle to prevent friction			

Hip Adduction Grades 1 and 0				
Supine lying position	Stand on the test side. One hand supports the ankle and other palpates the adductor muscle	Patient attemopt to adduct the hip	Bring your leg in (try it)	*Grade 1*: Examiner can palpate adductor muscle (contractile response) but no joint movement is visible
				Grade 0: No palpable contraction. No movement

Hip External Rotation Grades 5, 4 and 3				
Patient position	*Therapist position*	*Testing/procedure*	*Instruction*	*Result*
Short sitting position with trunk supported by placing hand on the couch	Sit on the low stool. Place one hand over the ankle just above the malleolus and other hand will counterforce over the lateral aspect of distal thigh	Patient externally rotates the hip	Do not let me to move your leg outside	*Grade 5*: Hold against end of range against maximal resistance
				Grade 4: Hold against end of range against moderate resistance
				Grade 3: Hold end positions without resistance

Hip External Rotation Grade 2				
Supine lying and test limb is in internal rotation.	Stand at the test side of the limb	Patient externally rotates the hip with one hand supporting the lateral hip	Roll your test limb out	*Grade 2*: Patient completes the external rotation

Hip External Rotation Grades 1 and 0				
Supine lying with test limb in internal rotation	Stand at the test side	Patient attempts to externally rotate the hip	Roll your leg out (try it)	*Grade 1*: Examiner can palpate only a contractile response but no joint movement is visible
				Grade 0: No palpable contraction. No movement.

Hip Internal Rotation Grades 5, 4 and 3				
Patient position	*Therapist position*	*Testing/procedure*	*Instruction*	*Result*
Short sitting position, arms may be kept on the couch for trunk support	Therapist sit on the low stool or in kneeling position	The limb should be placed at the end position of full inter-	Move your leg in towards the other one	*Grade 5*: Hold against end of range against

Contd.

Contd.

with one hand grasping the lateral surface of the anlkle just above the malleolus giving resistance as a medial directed force, i.e. inward and with other hand stabilizes the knee just distal to thigh offering lateral directed force	nal rotation for examiner for best test result.		Do not let me pull your leg inside	maximal resistance. *Grade 4*: Hold against end of range against moderate resistance *Grade 3*: Hold end positions without resistance

Hip Internal Rotation Grade 2

Supine lying position with test limb in partial external rotation.	Stand at the test side and palpate the gluteus medius and TFL	Patient will internally rotate the hip through the available range	Roll your legs inward towards the other leg	*Grade 2*: Patient completes the range of motion

Hip Internal Rotation Grades 1 and 0

Supine lying position with test limb in external rotation	Stand next to the test side of the patient	Patient will attempt to internally rotate the hip	Try to roll your test leg in	*Grade 1*: Examiner can palpate only a contractile res-ponse but no joint movement is visible *Grade 0:* No palpable contraction. No movement

Knee Flexion Grades 5, 4 and 3

Patient position	*Therapist position*	*Testing/procedure*	*Instruction*	*Result*
Prone lying with knee flexion about 45°	Stand at the test side of the patient at the level of hip. One hand is placed over the hamstring tendon and other hand gives resistance outward while grasping just above the malleolus	Patient flexes the knee in resistance	Bend your knee Hold it, do not let me push your leg down	*Grade 5*: Hold against end of range against maximal resistance *Grade 4*: Hold against end of range against moderate resistance *Grade 3*: Hold end positions without resistance

Knee Flexion Grade 2

Side lying position with test limb supported by examiner and non-test side is placed in slght flexion	Stand behind the patient at the hip level with one hand cradles the thigh to give support medially and other hand supports the leg just above the malleolus	Patient flexes the knee through the available range of motion	Bend your knee	*Grade 2*: Patient completes the range of motion in side lying position

Contd.

Contd.

Knee Flexion Grades 1 and 0

Prone lying with partial flexion of knee which is supported distally by the examiner	Standing next to the test limb at the knee level. One hand provides support to the lower leg just above the malleolus and with the other hand, palpate the hamstring tendon	Patient attempt to flex the knee	Bend your knee (try it)	*Grade 1*: Examiner can palpate only hamstring tendon contractile activity but no joint movement is visible *Grade 0*: No palpable contraction. No movement

Knee Extension Grades 5, 4 and 3

Patient position	*Therapist position*	*Testing/procedure*	*Instruction*	*Result*
Short sitting position with hands supporting the couch for trunk control	Standing at the side of the limb with one hand placed under the distal aspect of thigh and other hand counterforce the distal ankle just above the malleolus in downward direction	Patient should extend the knee through the available range of motion	Make your knee straight, hold it and do not bend it down	*Grade 5*: Hold against end of range against maximal resistance *Grade 4*: Hold against end of range against moderate resistance *Grade 3*: Hold end positions without resistance

Knee Extension Grade 2

Side lying position with the test limb placed upward and to maintain stability the lower limb is flexed. Test limb should be 90° flexed with hip fully extended	Stand behind the patient at the knee level. One arm may cradle around the under knee and with the other hand hold the leg above the malleolus	Patient should try to extend the k nee while therapist provides neither assistance nor resistance to the patient's voluntary movements	Straighten your knee	*Grade 2*: Patient completes the range of motion in side lying position

Knee Extension Grades 1 and 0

Supine lying position	Stand at the knee level near the test side. Place your 2–4 fingers to palpate the tendon of quadricep muscle and also the patellar tendon	Patient attempt to extend the knee	Try to tighten your kneecap	*Grade 1*: Examiner can palpate only contractile activity in the muscle through the ten-don but no joint movement is visi-ble *Grade 0*: No palpable contraction. No movement.

Contd.

Contd.

Ankle Plantar Flexion Grades 5, 4 and 3

Patient position	Therapist position	Testing/procedure	Instruction	Result
Standing position with the knee extended on the test side (use of only 1–2 finger for support)	Standing or sitting while watching the lateral view of the patient test limb	Patient will raise the heel from the floor through full range of plantar flexion	Stand on your legs now get up on to your toes, come down repeat it for 25 times	*Grade 5*: Patient successfully completed 25 heel rises through full range of motion without break in between
				Grade 4: Patient successfully completed 10–24 heel rises through full range of motion without break in between.
				Grade 3: Patient successfully completed 1–9 heel rises correctly wih no rest.

Ankle Plantar Flexion Grade 2

Stand on the test limb with knee extended with 2–4 finger support as assistance of table	Standing or sitting with the lateral view of patient fully visible of the test limb	Patient will attempt to raise the heel from the floor through full range of plantar flexion	Stand on your leg and try to stand on your toes. Repeat test for other leg	*Grade 2*: Patient just perform off the ground activity but cannot get up on to the toes

Ankle Plantar Flexion Grades 1 and 0

Prone lying with feet at the edge of the table	Stand at the test side in front of the table. Palpate the tendon of gastrocnemius and soleus (tendoachilles).	Patient will attempt to plantarflex the ankle.	Point your toe down	*Grade 1*: Examiner can palpate only contractile activity in the muscle through the tendon but no joint movement is visible
				Grade 0: No palpable contraction. No movement.

Ankle Dorsiflexion and Inversion Grades 5–0

Patient position	Therapist position	Testing/procedure	Instruction	Result
Short sitting position.	Sitting on the stool with the patient foot resting on the thigh of the therapist. One hand is contoured above the malleolus on the posterior aspect of the leg for the grades 5 and 4.	While keeping toes in relaxed position, patient dorsiflex ankle and invert the foot.	Bring your toes up and inward, hold it and do not let me pull it down	*Grade 5*: Complete full ROM and hold it against the maximal resistance.
				Grade 4: Complete full ROM against moderate resistance

Contd.

Contd.

	The hand providing resistance is cupped over the dorsal and medial aspect of the foot.			Grade 3: Complete full range of motion without resistance
				Grade 2: Complete only partial range of motion
				Grade 1: No joint movement only some contractile activity can be noted
				Grade 0: No palpable contraction

Plantar Flexion with Foot Eversion Grades 5–2

Patient position	Therapist position	Testing/procedure	Instruction	Result
Short sitting position with ankle in neutral position	Sitting on the stool placing one hand above the malleoli and other hand is contoured to give resistance over the dorsolateral aspect of the forefoot	Patient will evert the foot with depression over the first metatarsal head with some plantar flexion	Bring your foot down and out, hold it and do not let me to pull it in	Grade 5: Patient completes the full range of motion against maximal resistance
				Grade 4: Patient completes the full range of motion against moderate resistance
				Grade 3: Patient completes the full range of motion without resistance
				Grade 2: Patient completes the available range of motion partially eversion motion

Plantar Flexion with Foot Eversion Grades 1 and 0

Short sitting position	Sitting on a low stool and with the help of finger palpate the tendon of peroneus longus and brevis	Patient will attempt to plantarflex and evert the foot	Bring your foot down and out	Grade 1: Only contractile activity is felt. No motion occurs
				Grade 0: No motion, no contraction

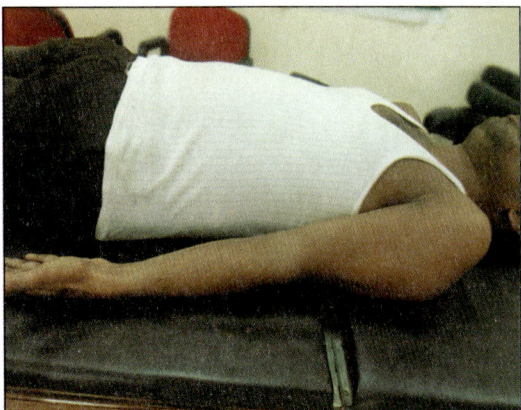 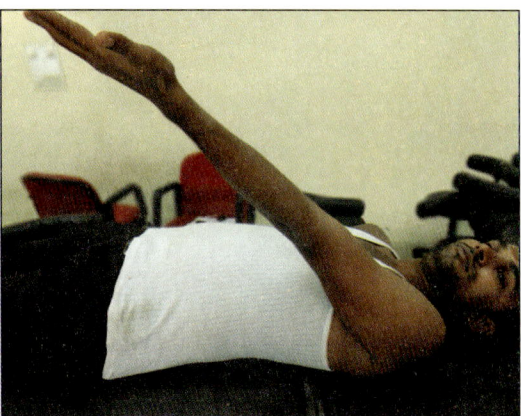

Grade 3: Shoulder flexion

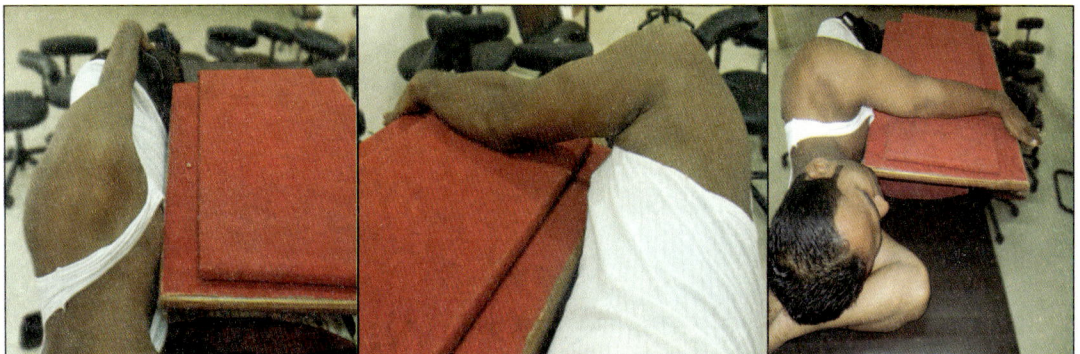

Grade 2: Shoulder flexion

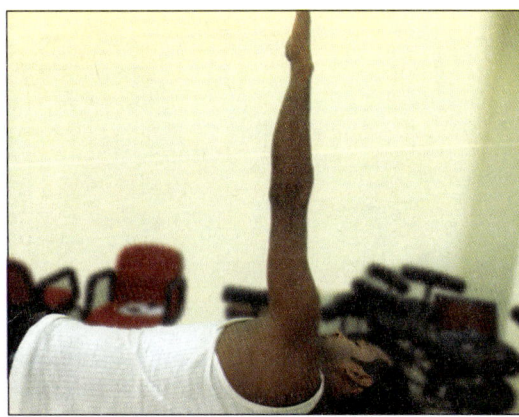 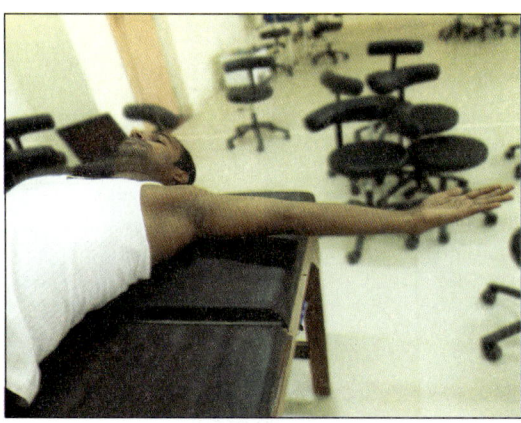

Grade 3: Shoulder abduction   **Grade 2:** Shoulder abduction

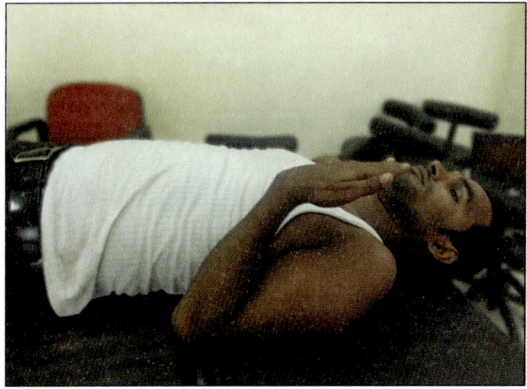

Grade 3: Hip flexion

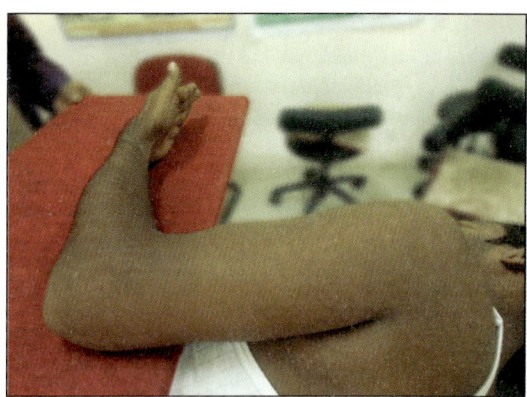

Grade 2: Elbow flexion

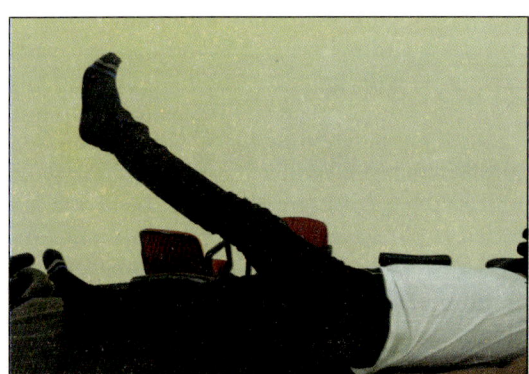

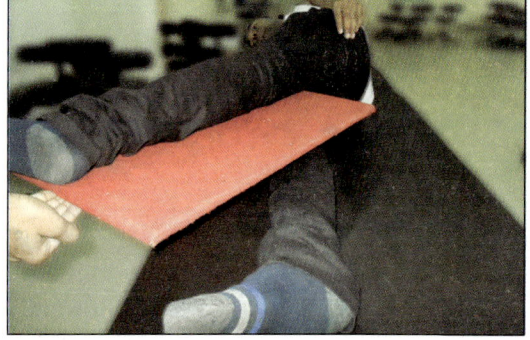

Grade 2: Hip flexion

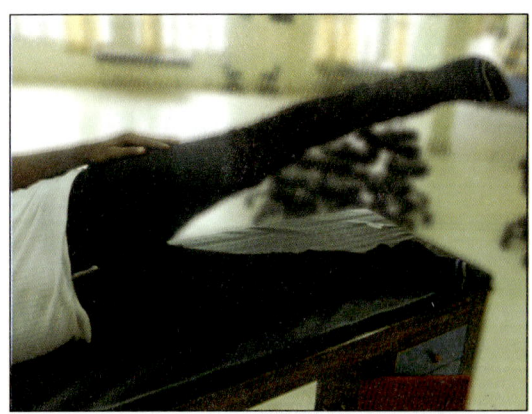

Grade 3: Hip abduction

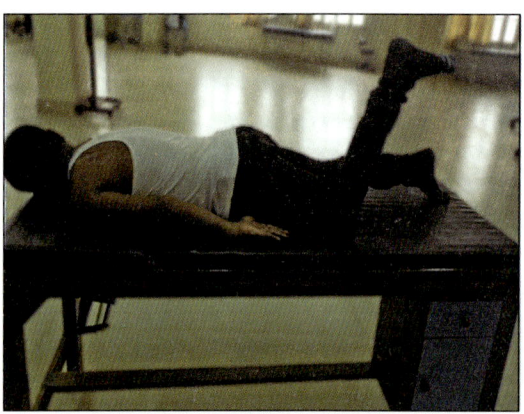

Grade 3: Knee flexion

Index

Abdominal reflex 32
Abduction or valgus stress test 72
Abstract thought 13
Acuity of vision 15
Adduction or varus stress test 72
ADL assessment 8, 47
Air bronchogram 121
Ankle dorsiflexion 60
Ankle dorsiflexion and inversion 161
Ankle jerk 37
Ankle plantar flexion 161
Antalgic gait 8, 42
Anterior Drawer test of ankle 74
Apex heart beat 94, 108
Apgar scoring 86
Apley's test 73, 74
Apprehension test 75
Approximation test 69
Apraxia 13
Assessment of edema 10
Assessment of higher function 12
Assessment of jugular venous pressure 107
Asymmetrical gait 44
Ataxic gait 45
Athetosis 9
Athrogenic gait 42
Auscultation of breath sounds 112
Auscultation of heart sounds 113
Auscultation skills 112
Axillary pulse 105

Balance and coordination 49
Balance test 7
Balint's syndrome 20
Barrel chest 108
Basics of electrocardiogram 122
Bathroom scale 147
Berg balance scale 7
Biceps jerk 35
Bladder and bowel assessment 46
Body mass index 147
Bowstring test 69
Brachial pulse 105
Brachioradialis jerk 35
Brainstem reflexes 90

Brudzinski's sign 68
Buccal pigmentation 97

Cardiac axis 127
Cardiac cycle 122
Cardiopulmonary assessment form 93
Cardiorespiratory assessment 93
Cardiothoracic ratio 120
Carotid pulse 105
Cerebellar ataxia 8
Cervical extension 61
Cervical lateral flexion 61
Cervical rotation 60
Chorea 9
Clonus 40
Clubbing of digits 100
Colli's horizontal suspension 88
Colli's vertical suspension 89
Colour vision 16
Concentric needle electrode 137
Conduction velocity 134
Congestive cardiac failure 121
Corneal arcus 99
Corneal reflex 21, 30
Cortical reactions 91
Cranial nerve assessment 14
Cranial nerve assessment 5
Cremastric reflex 33
Crude tests of hearing 21
CT scan 138

Deep reflexes 34
Demusset's sign 98
Development of milestones 91
Distraction test 75
Dorsalis pedis pulse 105
Double simultaneous stimulation 28
Drawer sign A 72
Drawer sign B 73
Drumstick-like fingers 100
Drunken sailor gait 8
Dysarthria 9
Dysphasia 9
Dysphonia 9
Dystonia 9

Edema 10, 101
Eithoven's triangle 124

Elbow extension 153
Elbow flexion 60, 152
Electrodiagnosis SD curve 130
Electromyography 136
El-Gon 53
Ely's test 71
Empty can test 77
Equinus gait 45
Examination of a chest radiograph 115
Examination of breathing pattern 109
Examination of chest mobility 110
Examination of chest shape and dimensions 108
Examination of cough 113
Examination of the distal pulses 103

Facial nerve 21
Fasiculation 9
Festinating gait 8
FG test 132
Field of vision 16
Finkelstein test 78
Foraminal compression test 74
Fundoscopy 17
Funnel chest 108

Gag reflex 32
Gait analysis 42
Gait assessment 42
Gapping test 69
Genslen's test 70
Gillet's test 70
Glasgow coma scale 5, 12
Glossopharyngeal nerve 23
Gluteus maximus gait 8
Golfer's elbow 78
Goniometry 53
Grades of dyspnea 109
Graphesthesia 28
Grimace 11

Hand to knee gait 45
Heart murmurs 95
Heart shadow 120
Hemiplegic gait 45
Hemochromatosis 97
Hepatojugular reflex 107
High stepping gait 8

Hip abduction 58, 156
Hip adduction 157
Hip extension 156
Hip external rotation 158
Hip flexion 59, 155
Hip internal rotation 158
Hip medical rotation 59
History 2
    present 3
    past 3
    medical 3
    personal 3
    marital 3
    family 3
    economic 3
    social 3
Hypoglossal nerve 24

Illingworth scale 87
Indurated edema 10, 101
Investigations 115
Involuntary movements 9

J sign 71
Jaw jerk 21
Joint kinesthetic sense 27
Joint position sense 26
Jugular venous pressure 94, 107

Kendall test 71
Knee extension 160
Knee flexion 59, 159
Knee jerk 35

Lachman test 72
Lasegue's test 67
Lateral epicondylitis 77
Level of consciousness 5
Lhermitt's test 68
Limb girth measurement of upper
    limb 65
Limb girth measurements 64
Limb length measurements 62
Lower lobe expansion 110

Magnetic resonance imaging 142
Malar flush 97
Manual muscle testing 148
Mcmurray test-A 73
Mcmurray test-B 73
Measurement of inversion and
    eversion 56
Measurement of range of motion 53
Medial epicondylitis 78
Mediastinal shift 102
Midbrain reaction 82
Midbrain reactions 91
Middle lobe expansion 110
Modified Ashworth scale 7, 39
Modified SLR test 68
Monopolar needle 137
Motor assessment 7
Motor examination 38

Muscle tightness 40
Musculoskeletal assessment 52
Myotomes 7

Need of diagnosis 1
Neer impingement test 76
Neonatal reflexes 81, 89
Nerve conduction velocity 134
Neurological assessment 4
Normal ECG 126

Objective assessment 1
Obstetrics and gynecology
    assessment 79
Oculomotoer apraxia 20
Olfactory nerve 15
One leg standing lumbar extention
    test 69
Optic ataxia 20
Optic nerve 15
Osler's nodules 99

P wave 126
Palpebral reflex 31
Parameters of gait 42
Parkinsonian gait 45
Parrot beak appearance 100
Pathological gaits 42
Patrick's or Faber's or figure-of four or
    Jansen's test 70
Pediatric assessment 81
Percussion 111
Peripheral cyanosis 98
Phalen's test 78
Pieper and Isbert reaction 89
Pigeon chest 108
Pitting type edema 11, 101
Plantar flexion with foot eversion 162
Plantar reflex 34
Polycythemia 98
Popliteal pulse 105
Posterior apprehension test 75
PR interval 127
Prone ante-rior drawer test 74
Prone anterior instability test 75
Prone knee bending test 68
Psychological assessment 48
Pupillary reflex 17, 30
Push or pull test 75

QRS complex 127
QT interval 129
Quadriceps jerk 35

Radial pulse 105
Recording of arterial blood pressure 106
Reflex examination 6, 30
Reflex maturation 88
Rinne test 22
Roos test 77

Sacral apex pressure 69
Schamroth's test 100
Scissor gait 8

Scissoring gait 45
Sensory assessment 5, 25
Short leg gait 45
Shoulder abduction 60, 150, 151
Shoulder extension 150
Shoulder external rotation 151
Shoulder flexion 60, 150
Shoulder internal rotation 152
Silhouette sign 120
Simultanagnosia 20
Six cardinal direction movements of
    eyeball 19
Slump test 67
Special tests in musculoskeletal
    assessment 67
Speed test 76
Spinal accessory nerve 23
Spinal level reflexes 90
Spinal reflexes 82
Spurling's test 74
ST segment 128
Stereognosis 27
Stoop's test 69
Subjective assessment 1, 2
Superficial reflexes 30
Symmetrial gait 43

T wave 129
TA jerk 36, 37
Tactile localization 27
Target heart rate 114
Tennis elbow 77
Testing of tone 38
Thomas test 71
Tibial pulse 105
Tics 9
Tinnel's sign 78
Tracheal shift 102
Trendelenburg sign 8
Trendelenburg's gait 45
Trendelenburg's test 71
Triceps jerk 35
Trigeminal nerve 19
Trigeminal neuralgia 21
Two point discrimination 28

Upper lobe expansion 110

Vagus nerve 23
Vestibulocochlear nerve 21
Visual field 16
Vocal fremitus 103
Vojta's reactions 87

Waddling gait 8
Weber test 22
Winding off 131
Wrist extension 154
Wrist flexion 153

Xanthelasma 99

Yergason's test 76